Writing SOAP Notes
Second Edition

Ginge Kettenbach, MS, PT
Clinical Education Coordinator
Christian Hospital Northeast–Northwest
and
Adjunct Assistant Professor
St. Louis University
St. Louis, Missouri

F. A. DAVIS COMPANY • Philadelphia

F. A. Davis Company
1915 Arch Street
Philadelphia, PA 19103

Printed in the United States of America

Last digit indicates print number: 10 9 8 7 6 5

Publisher, Allied Health: Jean-François Vilain
Developmental Editor: Crystal McNichol
Production Editor: Glenn L. Fechner
Cover Designer: Louis J. Forgione

As new scientific information becomes available through basic and clinical research, recommended treatments and drug therapies undergo changes. The author and publisher have done everything possible to make this book accurate, up to date, and in accord with accepted standards at the time of publication. The author, editors, and publisher are not responsible for errors or omissions or for consequences from application of the book, and make no warranty, expressed or implied, in regard to the contents of the book. Any practice described in this book should be applied by the reader in accordance with professional standards of care used in regard to the unique circumstances that may apply in each situation. The reader is advised always to check product information (package inserts) for changes and new information regarding dose and contraindications before administering any drug. Caution is especially urged when using new or infrequently ordered drugs.

Preface to the Second Edition

Healthcare has changed tremendously since the first edition of this workbook went to press. The length of stay in the hospital has shortened for all diagnoses. More care is given in the home, extended care facilities, subacute units, and outpatient centers. Less of the patient's care is given at the acute care hospital. Function has received an even greater emphasis in goal setting and the delivery of healthcare services. Hopefully, this edition reflects some of these changes. Time frames for goals were shortened on most patient types, and function was emphasized. A SOAP format for functional outcomes documentation is offered as well as the more traditional type of SOAP note.

Clinical education has also changed in the past few years. Models working toward greater efficiency have been put in place with the advent of assigning more than one student to a clinical instructor. Clinicians have had to become more efficient, and new practitioners step into a world in which they are expected to function more efficiently than did their predecessors. I have observed clinical instructors using this text to assist the students in remembering how or learning how to document better and more efficiently. A good background and practice in writing notes is important before the student or new practitioner enters the clinic.

Changes in this edition of the book include attempts at addressing the importance of documentation for the COTA and PTA. I also tried to add more occupational therapy and generic upper extremity examples and exercises. Students are asked to rewrite traditional SOAP notes into a functional outcomes SOAP format. The worksheets are also removable for those of you who would choose to grade them. The Appendices are all removable. Students can take either the Appendices or the entire text to the clinic. Professors can collect Appendix A on the first day of class if they find the students copying answers directly onto the worksheets. A chapter on documentation forms and computerized documentation has been added, as many facilities are experiencing changes toward both of these types of documentation.

I want to thank all of you who gave us feedback on the areas that needed more development in this text. An attempt was made to meet your needs. Please continue to give us feedback. Documentation must continue to change as healthcare changes; information from you on what is happening and needed is helpful.

Several people gave freely of their time in the development of this edition of *Writing SOAP Notes*. Linda Guth-Stangl proofread the entire text and gave excellent suggestions for improvement. Karen Christopher, Susan Ahmad, Lori Brown, Kim Robinson, and Louise Mattingly, my OT colleagues in the clinic, answered numerous questions and were willing to let me learn from their patient care notes. Charles Mead of CareCentric Solutions, Inc., taught me much of what I know about computerized documentation and gave me feedback on the final chapter. The F. A. Davis staff were encouraging as work was completed; their patience was tremendous at times.

As with the first edition, my children, Kristen and Kathryn, patiently shared their mom during vacation and evening time with this text. My husband, Gerry, also deserves much thanks. He continues to be a source of educational wisdom and always goes the extra mile to make sure I have the time I need to complete my work. His encouragement and patience are a constant source of energy and enlightenment.

Ginge Kettenbach

Preface to the First Edition

Documentation of patient care has gained much emphasis during the past few years. Medicare and other third-party payers have changed documentation from something which should be done well to something which *must* be done well if the healthcare provider is to survive. As clinicians have had to look at their own documentation skills and begin to self-evaluate, they have also faced the ongoing problems of teaching proper documentation skills to new employees and students. Productivity studies and the pressure to give quality care with efficiency continue to plague clinicians as our students enter the clinic.

This workbook was written to try to help with one of the most time-consuming aspects of clinical instruction: teaching documentation. As a faculty member, I tried lecturing on note writing, knowing that my fellow faculty members would ask the students to write notes for their classes and that my colleagues in the clinic would expect students to write notes. After giving a few hours of detailed lecture, I tried giving the students a note to write. The results were worrisome. Very few of the students could write a decent note. This workbook is a response to that need.

"Students have always learned to write notes in the clinic. The most we can do is to give them some basics." I was told this again and again by both clinicians and faculty. This workbook was written to give students the type of practice at note writing that they would normally get only very early in the clinical setting. Students were asked to decide which type of information belongs in which part of the note, to put various statements in order and under appropriate headings, and finally, to write the various parts of a SOAP note.

The following year, I let the clinicians be the final judges of the success of this workbook. "Tell me if you see any differences in the students' note writing skills this year. We tried something different." The clinicians *did* notice a difference. I also tested the students' note writing skills. Not every student note was perfect, but the information *was* categorized correctly, and the notes were all quite well organized.

As the years have passed, my original worksheets have become a workbook. It contains explanations of the relationship between writing SOAP notes and the problem-solving process the therapist experiences with each patient as well as detailed examples of the various parts of a note. Appendices, which can be detached and taken with the student to the clinic for quick reference, have been added. It is written on a simple level and can be used with early students who will eventually practice at either the therapist or assistant level.

It is hoped that this workbook will make the life of the clinical instructor as well as the work of the academic faculty simpler. I have played both roles and know that the problem of note writing is a difficult one for all involved. Most of all, I hope this workbook will help our new practitioners to make the quantum leap from the classroom to the clinic with a little more grace and ease.

In the early development of this workbook, I received much support from my ever-patient secretary, Annette AufderHeide. The faculty at St. Louis University who shared Annette's time with me also deserve special thanks. Four special people reviewed this workbook and gave me a tremendous amount of helpful feedback in its final revisions: Professor Susan B. O'Sullivan, MS, RPT, University of Lowell; Professor Heather Henager, MA, PT, Eastern Washington University; Professor Lynn S. Foord, PT, Simmons College; and Professor Thomas Schmitz, MS, PT, College of Physicians and Surgeons of Columbia University. Also, thanks to Professor Janice E. Toms, MEd, PT, Simmons College; Professor Lynn A. Colby, MS, BS, PT, Ohio State University; Professor Meryl R. Gersh, MMS, PT, Eastern Washington University; Professor Linda D. Crane, MMSc, PT, CCS, University of Miami; and Professor Cynthia Norkin, EdD, PT, College of Health and Human Services for their assistance.

Of course, much thanks goes to my family for all of their patience and time. My daughters, Kristen and Kathryn, have been supportive in their little ways, as they have literally grown up with this book. Cathy Kaiser, our friend, has given many extra hours of child care for the sake of this book. Gerry, my husband, has given me educational consultation and feedback that has been absolutely essential. Most of all, he has been a never-ending source of encouragement and support. Without these people, this workbook would remain in its original rough draft form.

Ginge Kettenbach

Contents

How to Use
This Book

This book was written to help new practitioners learn the skill of writing patient care notes. Like any other skill, writing notes takes practice. After each section of the note is discussed, an opportunity for practice is given in the worksheets at the end of the chapter. Several of the introductory chapters do not have worksheets because they cover prerequisite material needed for note writing and documentation in general.

Abbreviations

Chapter 3, "Using Abbreviations," introduces you to the abbreviations most commonly seen and/or used by therapists. The abbreviations listed for Hospital XYZ are acceptable for use throughout the rest of the workbook. If an abbreviation does not appear on the list, it is not to be used to complete the worksheets.

Medical Terminology

Worksheets are offered after a very brief discussion of medical terminology. These worksheets serve only as a review of your knowledge of medical terminology. They assume that you have previously studied medical terminology in depth. If you cannot complete these worksheets without difficulty, a review of medical terminology is suggested.

Successful Completion of the Worksheets

The first chapters will further explain problem solving and SOAP notes, why they are written, and what is meant by these terms. A careful reading of the text in each chapter will assist you both in successfully completing the worksheets and, ultimately, in successful note writing.

The benefits derived from completing the worksheets in this workbook depend upon the learner. If you are a novice at documentation, it is very important to complete each worksheet before referring to the answers in Appendix A. There are as many variations to note writing as there are practitioners. If your answers are not exactly the same as those provided, determine whether your answers would be considered acceptable and why the answers given in the book might or might not be preferable to your answers. By first completing the worksheets and then comparing your work, you will learn in the same manner in which learning takes place in the clinic. Individual practice and feedback have always proved to be the best methods of learning to write notes. If you are an experienced therapist, the text should prove to be worthwhile; you can use the worksheets as they prove to be of value to you.

Appendices

Appendix A contains the answers for the worksheets. The remaining appendices were written as references for you to use. It is suggested that you remove Appendices C and D from this book and take them with you to the clinic to assist you with note writing.

Appendix B includes a brief summary of the problem-solving process and its relationship to writing SOAP notes.

Appendix C is a summary of what is included in each part of the SOAP note. A description of the contents of interim notes and discharge summaries is also included.

Appendix D contains a summary of hints for effective writing to maximize reimbursement by third-party payers.

Appendix E contains a list of texts for further reading on topics covered in this workbook. It is assumed that new practitioners have access to a library to search for recent journal articles on assessment tools and documentation.

Appendix F gives one case written using three different methods of recording the same information in a SOAP format. The first method shows the information written in a traditional SOAP note format. In the second method, a flow sheet is used as a supplement to a SOAP note. In the third method, a flow sheet that is organized following the SOAP format is used instead of a traditional SOAP note.

Summary

The goal of this workbook is to provide the basic skills needed to write a SOAP note. Appendices are provided for reference as you enter the clinic. They may be detached for use in the clinic. A list of abbreviations to be used while completing the worksheets is included in Chapter 3. A review of medical terminology is provided in Chapter 4.

This book will not teach you to make all of the decisions necessary to assess and treat a patient. In each of the cases used in the worksheets, you will be given assistance in making decisions regarding setting goals or setting up a treatment plan. However, it is suggested that you take advantage of the examples of problem solving that are given to you as you complete the worksheets. In completing the worksheets, you are given the rationale behind decisions, step by step, as they would be made by an experienced clinician. This is the type of problem solving that you will be expected to perform as you assess and treat patients while performing patient care as a professional.

Introduction to SOAP Notes **1**

Each day in the clinic, physical and occupational therapists, physical therapist assistants, occupational therapy assistants, and many other healthcare professionals document what they do with patients. One of the methods they use is a form of patient care note called a SOAP note. The SOAP format for writing notes is not the only method used in therapy clinics. However, it is very commonly used throughout the country. It would be rare for a therapist or assistant not to encounter the SOAP note format, or one of its variations, during his or her career as a student and later as a practicing therapist.

What SOAP Means

SOAP is an acronym. Each of the letters in SOAP stands for the name of a section of the patient note. The patient note is divided as follows:

S stands for Subjective.
O stands for Objective.
A stands for Assessment.
P stands for Plan.

In many facilities, a fifth section, the Problem, is included before the S portion of the note.

Types of Notes

During the course of a patient's care, the patient is initially assessed, reassessed constantly, and finally assessed upon discharge from the therapist's care. Each of these types of assessment results in a type of SOAP note. An **initial** note is written after the initial patient assessment. An **interim,** or **progress,** note is written periodically, reporting the results of reassessment. A **discharge** note is written at the time that therapy is discontinued.

The Origin of SOAP Notes

The SOAP note format was introduced by Dr. Lawrence Weed as a part of a system of organizing the medical record called the problem-oriented medical record (POMR). The POMR has one list

4 of patient problems in the front of the chart, and each healthcare practitioner writes a separate SOAP note to address each of the patient's problems. Many facilities never use the POMR; rather, they use some other type of medical record format. Other facilities use a somewhat adapted POMR format. In any case, one contribution that clearly came from the POMR is a widespread use of the SOAP note format.

Professionals in many medical and allied health fields have adapted the original SOAP format of note writing into a practical tool that is used for documentation today. Unfortunately, each field and each facility has its own variation of the SOAP note. As you enter each clinical facility during your training and later during your professional practice, you will adapt your method of note writing to conform with the variation used by the facility. This workbook will teach you a comprehensive method of writing SOAP notes that can be adapted to meet the requirements and needs of any facility.

Functional Outcomes Reporting in a SOAP Format

Some facilities are adapting the traditional SOAP format into a SOAP format called functional outcomes reporting. These facilities write SOAP notes that emphasize and discuss the patient's functional status and set goals and treatment to improve function only. Those who use this type of note format do so to emphasize the true goal of therapy: to improve patient function. Many believe that functional outcomes reporting will be the format used for note writing in the future. However, many differences exist between the functional outcomes formats of notes used in each facility. Since the SOAP format is compatible with functional outcomes reporting, learning the SOAP format can help you prepare for note writing now and in the future. Differences between the traditional SOAP note format and the functional outcomes SOAP note format will be discussed in each chapter of this book.

The Purposes of Documentation

All healthcare professionals document their findings for several reasons:

1. Notes record what the therapist does to manage the individual patient's case. The rights of the therapist and the patient are protected should any question occur in the future regarding the care provided to the patient. SOAP notes are considered legal documents, as are all parts of the medical record.

2. A SOAP note is a method of communicating with the patient's physician and other healthcare professionals, including other therapists and therapist assistants. The note communicates the results of the patient interview, the objective measurements done, and the therapist's assessment of the patient's condition. It communicates the therapist's (and patient's) goals for the patient and the plan for treatment. The goal of such communication is to provide consistency between the services provided by various healthcare professionals.

   In the case of absence from the clinic, a good SOAP note can help a therapist communicate with other therapists or assistants who may provide substitute care for his or her patients during the absence. In a rehabilitation center, school setting, or other settings using the rehabilitation team approach, the therapist's goals and the patient's level of function can be communicated to the other professionals involved in the patient's care. Professionals providing services after the patient is discharged from one therapist's care may find the therapist's notes to be very valuable in providing good follow-up treatment.

3. Third-party payers, such as Medicare reviewers and representatives from insurance companies, make decisions about reimbursement based on therapy notes. These decisions can be greatly influenced by the quality and completeness of the note.

4. Within the hospital and other types of facilities, patient charts are reviewed. Decisions on whether the patient is ready to be discharged are made based, in part, on the notes written by the therapist or assistant.

5. Using the SOAP method of writing notes helps the therapist to organize the thought processes involved in patient care. By thinking in an organized manner, the therapist can better make decisions regarding patient care. Thus, the SOAP note is an excellent method of structuring thinking for problem solving.

6. A SOAP note can be used for quality assurance and improvement purposes. Certain criteria are set to indicate whether quality care is occurring. Within a limited time frame, the SOAP notes from all patients with a certain diagnosis can be assessed to see whether the preset criteria have been met.

7. SOAP notes can be used in research. As with quality assurance, certain criteria are initially set for the type of patient to be included, data to be taken, and so forth. Data from the notes can be gathered and conclusions drawn about the type of patient and/or the type of treatment provided.

As a therapist or therapist assistant, it is important to realize that documentation is as integral a part of the patient care process as the assessment or treatment of the patient. Each day a significant portion of time is spent by a therapist or assistant in documenting what we do and why.

The Relationship of SOAP Notes to the Decision-Making Process

As mentioned previously, using SOAP notes helps the therapist organize and plan quality patient care. Following the SOAP note format presented in this workbook does not assure good problem-solving skills; however, it does provide a structure within which good problem solving will more likely occur. During an initial session with the patient, the process of assessment and decision making occurs in the following manner:

1. The therapist reads the patient's chart (medical record) or referral (if either is available). Test results such as x-ray examinations and laboratory findings as well as the physician's impression of the patient's problem can assist in planning the patient interview and identifying measurements to be performed.

    The results from this portion of the process are stated in the section called **Problem** or **Diagnosis.**

2. The therapist then interviews the patient. Information is gathered regarding the patient's history, complaints, home situation, and goals for therapy.

    The subjective information thus gathered comprises the **Subjective,** or **S,** portion of the note.

3. From the information gathered from the medical record and the patient, the therapist plans the objective measurements to be performed. Then the planned measurements are completed.

    The results of these measurements performed are recorded in the **Objective,** or **O,** portion of the note.

4. Once the therapist has completed the interview and measurement process, she or he interprets the information recorded and identifies factors that are not within normal limits for people in the same age range as the patient. From these factors, the therapist formulates a list of the patient's problems, including functional limitations and impairments.

    The patient's problems are recorded in a section of the note called **Functional Limitations** or the **Problem List,** depending on the facility and what it includes in this section. Functional Limitations or the Problem List is part of the **Assessment,** or **A,** portion of the note.

5. After formulating a list of the patient's functional limitations or problems, the therapist and the patient together establish goals that correspond to the patient's functional limitations or problems. The first set of goals, or functional outcomes, states the final result of therapy, or the extent to which each of the patient's functional limitations or problems should be resolved following a program of therapeutic intervention.

The goals stating the intended outcomes of therapy are called **Functional Outcomes** or **Long Term Goals.** The Functional Outcomes or Long Term Goals are also included in the **Assessment,** or **A,** portion of the note.

6. After the Functional Outcomes or Long Term Goals are established, the therapist and patient consider what can be achieved within a short period of time (usually by the time a progress note is written, that is, if the patient is to be in the therapist's care long enough for a progress note to be written). Goals are then set for this short period of time.

The goals stating what can be achieved in a short period of time are called **Short Term Goals.** The Short Term Goals are written into the **Assessment,** or **A,** portion of the note.

7. Once the therapist and the patient together make decisions regarding the anticipated outcomes or goals of treatment, the therapist formulates impressions of the patient's problems and conditions. Justifications of unusual goals or patient parameters that could not be measured or cannot be treated are listed.

The therapist's **Summary** and/or **Impressions** are listed in the **Assessment,** or **A,** part of the note.

8. After setting goals with the patient, the therapist outlines a treatment plan to achieve them. The plan for treatment is listed as the **Plan,** or **P,** part of the note.

Documentation of Healthcare Delivery by the PTA or COTA

The PTA or COTA often reads the initial documentation of the patient's condition, goals, and care plan and is expected to follow the plan as outlined by the therapist in the initial patient note. After the patient has been seen by the PTA or COTA for a period of time (this period of time varies according to the policies of each facility and state law), the PTA or COTA must write an interim note documenting any changes in the patient's status that have occurred since the therapist's initial note was written. Also, after discussion of the patient's condition, goals, and treatment with the therapist, the assistant rewrites or responds to the previously written short term goals and revises the patient's treatment plan accordingly. In most facilities, the therapist then cosigns the assistant's notes, indicating agreement with what was documented in the notes. (Once again, this depends on the facility's policies and state law.)

It is extremely important for both therapists and assistants to remember the importance of the role of assistants in documenting patient care. Assistants can develop the skill to participate as fully in documentation of patient care as they do in delivering patient care. With healthcare delivery changing, assisting with documentation is a valuable role for the assistant, and documentation skills are as crucial to the assistant as they are to the therapist. Therefore, physical therapist assistant and occupational therapy assistant students are encouraged to take full advantage of the skills to be learned from this workbook.

Some of the notes written in the worksheets are examples of initial patient care notes. Although it is acknowledged that the assistant will not write an initial note in the clinic, the same skills used to write initial notes are used to write interim notes. Therefore, assistant students are encouraged to take advantage of the opportunities to write all of the sample notes in all of the worksheets. If it is helpful, think of the examples of initial notes as interims during which the therapist and assistant worked together to perform certain patient assessments and talked together about setting or resetting goals. This type of situation could occur in your future practice, with the therapist asking the assistant to write the note and the therapist then cosigning the note. Each facility differs in its use of assistants in both occupational and physical therapy. However, no matter what the specific details of the assistant's role are, it is clear that assistants need good documentation skills.

Summary

The SOAP note is one of the more commonly used forms of note writing. The SOAP format lends itself well to writing an initial note, as well as to writing interim notes and a discharge summary for each patient seen in therapy. It is probably the most comprehensive form of documentation encountered by most practitioners. Dr. Lawrence Weed's POMR format contained the origins of the SOAP note format that is more commonly used today.

Documentation has many purposes, from assuring quality care to communication to discharge planning. It has become very important in a healthcare atmosphere that includes lawsuits and the need of third-party payers to obtain clear and accurate information. The SOAP method of writing notes serves as a guide to thinking through problems, demonstrating accountability for quality patient care, and documenting patient care. All are needed as the new practitioner enters the clinic.

2 Writing in a Medical Record

The writing style used in medical notes at most clinical facilities differs from the style most students are accustomed to using when writing papers, reports, and so forth. Writing in patient charts or files requires using medical abbreviations and terminology and emphasizes brevity. The following guidelines are provided to assist you in becoming accustomed to writing in a medical record.

Accuracy

NEVER record falsely, exaggerate, or make up data. SOAP notes are part of a permanent, legal document. Incorrect spelling, grammar, and punctuation can be misleading. Objective information should be stated in a factual manner.

Keep information objective. Criticisms of other staff members and/or complaints about working conditions should not be included in the patient note. The note is about the patient and not about the healthcare provider.

Brevity

Information should be stated concisely. Use short, succinct sentences. Avoid long-winded statements. Also avoid strings of short clauses connected by "and." It is permissible to use sentence fragments or outline form at some facilities. Whatever style is used, it is important to be consistent in style to avoid confusion and to comply with the policies of the facility or practice setting.

EXAMPLE

BRIEF
Pt. amb 10 ft. in // bars indep. but required min assist of 1 to turn around in // bars. Sit↔stand from w/c indep. using // bars for support.

LONG AND WINDY
Once the patient wheeled up to the // bars and positioned himself in front of the // bars, he locked his w/c, raised the foot plates, and scooted forward from the seat of

the chair. He then gripped the // bars with his hands and on the count of 3 was able to pull himself up to a standing position without any assist. from the therapist. Once standing, he was able to ambulate by positioning his arms forward and then taking steps. He could lead with either right or left foot. Upon turning in the // bars, he was unable to let go with one arm to pivot his body around. Therapist had to give some support until the patient was turned around and both arms were back on the // bars.

Abbreviations can help with brevity. Abbreviations used should be from the accepted list of the facility at which you practice. During your orientation to the facility, you should ask for a copy of that facility's standard list of abbreviations.

Brevity can also be overdone. Enough information must be present to get ideas across. Almost every S and O statement contains a verb (or some sort of punctuation to replace a verb; see ''Punctuation'' below).

Clarity

The wording of SOAP notes should be such that the meaning is immediately clear to the reader. Sudden shifts in tense from past to present should be avoided.

EXAMPLE

Incorrect: Pt. stated she lived alone. Describes 5 steps $\bar{s}$ hand railing at entry of her 1-story house. Denied previous use of assistive device.

Correct: States lives alone. Describes 5 steps $\bar{s}$ hand railing at entry of her 1-story house. Denies previous use of assistive device.

Avoid vague terminology.

EXAMPLE

VAGUE
''ROM is ↑''
''feeling better''
''amb $\bar{c}$ some assist.''

CLEAR
''Ⓡ shoulder flexion AROM is ↑ to 0–70°''
''Pt. states she knows she is feeling better indicated by her ability to perform light housekeeping tasks for ~2 hrs. $\bar{a}$ tiring.''
''Pt. amb $\bar{c}$ walker NWB Ⓛ LE for ~20 ft × 2 $\bar{c}$ min +1 assist.''

It is important for handwriting to be legible. The purpose of writing notes is defeated if the notes cannot be easily read.

Using abbreviations that are standard to the facility is absolutely essential to assure clarity in note writing. Terminology used within a rehabilitation department, such as ''minimal assistance,'' should be well defined and used in a consistent manner by all therapists in the department.

Examples of Errors in Accuracy, Brevity, and Clarity

INCORRECT: Pt. was unable to perform activity due to *muscle absence.* (inaccurate and unclear)
CORRECT: . . . due to *muscle paralysis.*
INCORRECT: *Watch for* return of *absent muscles.* (unclear and inaccurate)
CORRECT: *Reassess prn* for *motor return.*

10

INCORRECT: Pt. is *sore*. (too brief; unclear)
CORRECT: Pt. is *sensitive to touch*.
INCORRECT: Pt. *didn't have any tightness*. (wordy; unclear)
CORRECT: *No ROM limitations* noted.
INCORRECT: *Had his* Ⓡ *leg cut off because of circulation problems*. (wordy)
CORRECT: Ⓡ *LE amputation 2° to PVD*.
INCORRECT: Pt. was unable to wiggle toes *when asked to*. (wordy)
CORRECT: Pt. was unable to wiggle toes *upon request*.
INCORRECT: Assessment *was* incomplete *because of* pt. confusion (wordy)
CORRECT: Assessment incomplete *2° to* pt. confusion.

Punctuation

HYPHEN (-)

Hyphens should be avoided in notes because they can be confused with the minus signs used in muscle grades or negatives (as in SLR: − on R). One exception is the common use of a hyphen instead of the word through (as in <u>AROM:</u> 0–48°).

SEMICOLON (;)

Instead of overusing "states" in the subjective part of the note, a semicolon can be used to connect two related statements.

EXAMPLE

Instead of "States position of comfort for sleep is on Ⓡ side. States pain does not awaken pt. at night . . . ," you could say "States position of comfort for sleep is on Ⓡ side; pain does not awaken pt. at night."

COLON (:)

A colon can be used instead of "is."

EXAMPLE

Instead of "AROM Ⓡ shoulder flexion is 0–90°," you could say "AROM Ⓡ shoulder flexion: 0–90°."

Correcting Errors

"Wite out" (correction fluid) should *not* be used on a medical record. Trying to destroy or attempting to obliterate information makes it look as if the health professional is trying to "cover up" malpractice. The proper method of correcting a mistake made in charting is to put a line through the error, write "(error)" above the mistake, date it, and initial it.

EXAMPLE

Correct:
(error)vkk 2/28/94
~~some~~ min +1 assist.

Signing Your Notes

You should sign every entry that you make into the medical record. All notes should be signed with your legal signature (your last name and legal first name or initials). No nicknames should be used.

Initials should follow your name indicating your status as a therapist or therapist assistant.

EXAMPLE

Sue Brown, PT or James Smith, PTA

Maryann Jones, OTR or Barbara McDonald, COTA

In some facilities, there is a custom of using additional initials prior to PT or PTA (L, P, or R). The American Physical Therapy Association advocates the use of PT or PTA only. The American Occupational Association advocates the use of OTR or COTA. In some clinics, students sign their notes SPT or SPTA, OTS or OTAS. Others ask the student to sign his or her name only. In either case, the signature of a student should *always* be followed by a slash and then the signature of the supervising therapist.

EXAMPLE

Gene White, SPT/Sue Brown, PT

Peter Maxwell, OTS/Maryann Jones, OTR

Referring to Yourself

Notes discuss the patient and not the therapist.

EXAMPLE

Incorrect: I helped this patient transfer $\bar{c}$ min assist. from his w/c to the plinth.

Correct: Pt. transferred $\bar{c}$ min assist. w/c$\leftrightarrow$plinth.

If for some reason a therapist must make reference to himself or herself, most facilities prefer that the reference be made in the third person as "therapist" or "physical therapist" or "occupational therapist."

EXAMPLE

Pt. states therapist should be putting his shoes on for him like his family does at home.

Blank or Empty Lines

Lines should not be left between one entry and another, nor should empty lines be left within a single entry. Empty lines are areas in which another person could falsify information already charted. Adding even one word, such as "not," to a note can completely change the meaning of the note's content.

Writing Orders in a Chart

When a physician gives an order to a therapist, the therapist is the professional responsible for writing it in the chart. In writing an order in the chart, the following format is standard in most facilities:

> date/time/order
> > v.o. physician's name/therapist's signature, OTR (or PT)

EXAMPLE

12-24-95/10:50/Pt. may be FWB in PT
v.o. Dr. Ache/Sue Brown, PT

Once the order is written by the therapist in the chart, the physician cosigns the order the next time he or she sees the chart or as soon as possible thereafter.

Summary

In summary, medical writing should be brief, accurate, and clear. Errors should be corrected, *not* erased or covered with correction fluid. You should use your legal signature as you would on any legal document. If you follow these guidelines and apply them throughout the exercises in this book, with time you will develop a good medical writing style that you will use daily as you practice in the clinic.

Using Abbreviations 3

Abbreviations are used as a time and space saver while writing notes. In order to ensure that everyone in the hospital can understand what has been written in the chart by others, most medical facilities have a list of approved abbreviations, and these are the *only* abbreviations that should be used in a medical record in that particular facility. This list of abbreviations is approved by the medical records department of each facility. The list of acceptable abbreviations varies from one facility to the next, particularly terminology specific to allied health fields such as physical and occupational therapy.

The list of abbreviations that follows will be used as the approved list for all of the worksheets in this book. It is a compilation of the most common abbreviations used by over 13 different healthcare facilities. Any abbreviations *not* on this list will be considered unacceptable for these worksheets. As you begin to write notes during your time in the clinic, please remember that the list of acceptable abbreviations for your clinical facility must be used. During orientation to any clinical facility in which you practice, you should ask about the location of the approved abbreviations list and become particularly familiar with the abbreviations used frequently by the facility. For further reference on abbreviations, see Appendix E.

Approved Abbreviations and Symbols for Hospital XYZ

A:	assessment
AAROM	active assistive range of motion
abd	abduction
ac	before meals
AC joints	acromioclavicular joints
ACTH	adrenocorticotrophic hormone
add	adduction
ADL	activities of daily living
ad lib	at discretion
adm	admission
AE	above elbow
AFO	ankle foot orthosis
AIDS	autoimmune deficiency syndrome
AIIS	anterior inferior iliac spine
AJ	ankle jerk

14

AK	above knee
a.m.	morning
AMA	against medical advice
amb	ambulation, ambulating, ambulated, ambulate, ambulates
ant	anterior
AP	anterior-posterior
AROM	active range of motion
ASA	aspirin
ASAP	as soon as possible
ASHD	arteriosclerotic heart disease
ASIS	anterior superior iliac spine
assist.	assistance, assistive
B/S	bedside
BE	below elbow
bid	twice a day
bilat.	bilateral, bilaterally
BK	below knee
BM	bowel movement
BP	blood pressure
bpm	beats per minute
BRP	bathroom privileges
BUN	blood urea nitrogen (blood test)
C	Centigrade
C & S	culture and sensitivity
CA	cancer, carcinoma
CABG	coronary artery bypass graft
CAD	coronary artery disease
cal	calories
CBC	complete blood count
CBI	closed brain injury
CBS	chronic brain syndrome
CC, C/C	chief complaint
cc	cubic centimeter
CHF	congestive heart failure
cm	centimeter
CNS	central nervous system
c/o	complains of
CO$_2$	carbon dioxide
COLD	chronic obstructive lung disease
cont.	continue
COPD	chronic obstructive pulmonary disease
COTA	certified occupational therapy assistant
CP	cerebral palsy
CPR	cardiopulmonary resuscitation
CSF	cerebral spinal fluid
CV	cardiovascular
CVA	cerebrovascular accident
CWI	crutch walking instructions
Cysto	cystoscopic examination
dept.	department
DIP	distal interphalangeal joint

D/C	discontinued or discharged
DM	diabetes mellitus
DO	doctor of osteopathy
DTR	deep tendon reflex
Dx	diagnosis
ECF	extended care facility
ECG, EKG	electrocardiogram
EEG	electroencephalogram
EENT	ear, eyes, nose, throat
EMG	electromyogram, electromyography
E.R.	emergency room
eval.	evaluation
ext.	extension
F	fair (muscle strength, balance)
FBS	fasting blood sugar
FH	family history
flex	flexion
ft.	foot, feet (the measurement, not the body part)
FUO	fever, unknown origin
FWB	full weight bearing
fx	fracture
G	good (muscle strength, balance)
GB	gallbladder
GI	gastrointestinal
gm	gram
GYN	gynecology
h, hr.	hour
H & H, H/H	hematocrit and hemoglobin
H & P	history and physical
HA, H/A	headache
Hb, Hgb	hemoglobin
HCVD	hypertensive cardiovascular disease
HEENT	head, ear, eyes, nose, throat
HEP	home exercise program
HI	head injury
HIV	human immunodeficiency virus
HNP	herniated nucleus pulposus
HOB	head of bed
HR	heart rate
hr.	hour
hs	at bedtime
ht.	height
Ht	hematocrit
Htn	hypertension
Hx	history
I & O	intake and output
ICU	intensive care unit
IM	intramuscular
imp.	impression

16

in.	inches
indep	independent
inf	inferior
IV	intravenous
kcal	kilocalories
kg	kilogram
KJ	knee jerk
KUB	kidney, ureter, bladder
L, l.	liter
Ⓛ	left
lb.	pound
LBP	low back pain
LE	lower extremity
LOC	loss of consciousness
LP	lumbar puncture
m	meter
max	maximal
MD	medical doctor; doctor of medicine
MED	minimal erythemal dose
Meds.	medications
MFT	muscle function test
mg	milligram
MI	myocardial infarction
min	minimal
min.	minutes
ml	milliliter
mm	millimeter
MMT	manual muscle test
mo.	month
mod	moderate
MP, MCP	metacarpalphalangeal
MS	multiple sclerosis
N	normal (muscle strength)
NDT	neurodevelopmental treatment
neg.	negative
N.H.	nursing home
noc	night, at night
npo	nothing by mouth
NSR	normal sinus rhythm
NWB	non-weight-bearing
O:	objective
OB	obstetrics
OBS	organic brain syndrome
od	once daily
O.P.	outpatient
O.R.	operating room
ORIF	open reduction, internal fixation
OT	occupational therapy, occupational therapist

OTR	occupational therapist (used to follow official signature of the occupational therapist)
oz.	ounce
P	poor (muscle strength, balance)
P:	plan (treatment plan)
P.A.	physician's assistant
PA	posterior/anterior
para	paraplegia
pc	after meals
per	by/through
per os, p.o.	by mouth
PERRLA	pupils, equal, round, reactive to light and accommodation
P.H.	past history
p.m.	afternoon
PNF	proprioceptive neuromuscular facilitation
PNI	peripheral nerve injury
POMR	problem-oriented medical record
pos.	positive
poss	possible
post	posterior
post-op	after surgery (operation)
PRE	progressive resistive exercise
pre-op	before surgery (operation)
prn	whenever necessary
PROM	passive range of motion
PSIS	posterior superior iliac spine
PT	physical therapy, physical therapist (used after therapist's signature; varies from facility to facility)
PT/PTT	protime/prothrombine time
Pt., pt.	patient
PTA	physical therapist assistant
PTA	prior to admission
PTB	patellar tendon bearing
PVD	peripheral vascular disease
PWB	partial weight bearing
q	every
qd	every day
qh	every hour
qid	four times a day
qn	every night
qt.	quart
®	right
RA	rheumatoid arthritis
RBC	red blood cell count
R.D.	registered dietician
re:	regarding
rehab	rehabilitation
reps	repetitions
resp	respiratory, respiration
RN	registered nurse
R/O	rule out (In order to make a good diagnosis, the physician will try to rule the disease/condition named out; if he or she cannot, this will become the diagnosis.)

18

ROM	range of motion	
ROS	review of systems	
RROM	resistive range of motion	
R.T.	respiratory therapist, respiratory therapy	
Rx	treatment, prescription, therapy	
SACH	solid ankle cushion heel	
SCI	spinal cord injury	
SC joint	sternoclavicular joint	
sec.	seconds	
SED	suberythemal dose	
sig	directions for use, give as follows, let it be labeled	
SI(J)	sacroiliac (joint)	
SLE	systemic lupus erythematosus	
SLR	straight leg raise	
SNF	skilled nursing facility	
SOAP	subjective, objective, assessment, plan	
SOB	shortness of breath	
S/P	status post (example: S/P Ⓛ hip fx means Pt. fx her hip in the recent past)	
spec	specimen	
stat.	immediately, at once	
Sx	symptoms	
T	trace (muscle strength)	
tab	tablet	
TB	tuberculosis	
tbsp.	tablespoon	
TENS, TNS	transcutaneous electrical nerve stimulator	
THR	total hip replacement	
TIA	transient ischemic attack	
tid	three times daily	
TKR	total knee replacement	
TM(J)	temporomandibular (joint)	
TNR	tonic neck reflex (also ATNR, STNR)	
t.o.	telephone order	
TPR	temperature, pulse & respiration	
tsp.	teaspoon	
TUR	transurethral resection	
UA	urine analysis	
UE	upper extremity	
UMN	upper motor neuron	
URI	upper respiratory infection	
US	ultrasound	
UTI	urinary tract infection	
UV	ultraviolet	
VD	venereal disease	
v.o.	verbal orders (example: v.o. Dr. Smith/your signature)	
vol.	volume	
v.s.	vital signs	
w/c	wheelchair	
W/cm²	watts per square centimeter	
WBC	white blood cell count	

wk.	week
WNL	within normal limits
wt.	weight
x	number of times performed ($\times 2$ = twice, $\times 3$ = 3 times)
y/o or y.o.	years old
yd.	yard
yr.	year
+1, +2	assistance (assistance of 1 person given; also written "assistance of 1") (Examples: amb . . . $\bar{c}$ min + 1 assist., or amb . . . $\bar{c}$ +1 min assist., or amb . . . $\bar{c}$ min assist. of 1)
♂	male
♀	female
↓	down, downward, decrease, diminished
↑	up, upward, increase, augmented
//	parallel or parallel bars (also written // bars)
$\bar{c}$	with
$\bar{s}$	without
$\bar{p}$	after
$\bar{a}$	before
~ **or** ≈	approximately
@	at (this symbol is not exclusively used for at)
△	change
>	greater than
<	less than
=	equals
+	plus, positive (positive also abbreviated pos.)
−	minus, negative (negative also abbreviated neg.)
#	number (#1 = number 1), pounds (5# wt. = 5 pound weight; also abbreviated lbs.)
/	per
%	percent
+, &, et.	and
↔, ⇌, ⇆	to and from
→	to, progressing toward, approaching
1°	primary
2°	secondary, secondary to

Using Abbreviations: Examples

The following are examples of the use of abbreviations in medical records.

1. In the doctor's notes, you may find the following: Pt. has hx of Htn, ASHD, CHF, MI in 1993, TIA in 1994.

Translation: The patient has a history of hypertension, arteriosclerotic heart disease, congestive heart failure, myocardial infarction in 1993, transient ischemic attack in 1994.

2. Orders written in the chart:
   Up ad lib
   ASA q 4 hrs.
   BRP prn
   NPO $\bar{p}$ midnight
   v.o. Dr. Smith/Janice Jones, OTR

Translation:
Up at discretion (patient's discretion)
Aspirin every 4 hours
Bathroom privileges when necessary
Nothing by mouth after midnight
Verbal order given by Dr. Smith to Janice Jones, occupational therapist

20

3. In PT note: Rx: AROM Ⓡ ankle bid

Translation: Treatment: Active range of motion right ankle twice per day.

4. In chart in doctor's initial note: imp: COPD; R/O lung CA

Translation: Impression: Chronic obstructive pulmonary disease; rule out lung cancer.

5. Physician's orders:
    record I & O
    all meds per IV
    NPO
    transfer pt. to ICU

Translation:
Record intake and output
All medications through intravenous (tube)
Nothing by mouth
Transfer patient to the intensive care unit.

You will be expected to be able to both interpret and use abbreviations in the medical record. You will encounter most of the abbreviations listed in this chapter when you practice in the clinic. Any time you write a note, you will be expected to use abbreviations properly.

Using Abbreviations: WORKSHEET 1

Translate each phrase or sentence written with abbreviations into a full English phrase or sentence. Translate each sentence or phrase written in English into a sentence or phrase written with abbreviations.

1. Physician's orders:
   to PT per w/c
   turn Pt. qh

   Translation:
   _____
   _____
   _____

2. In chart:
   Dx: RA; R/O SLE.

   Translation:
   _____
   _____

3. In PT note:
   Treatment: once per day, activities of daily living training, ultrasound at 1.0 to 1.5 watts per centimeter squared to anterior superior aspect of right knee for 5 minutes.

   Translation:
   _____
   _____
   _____

4. In OT or PT note:
   c/o SOB $\overline{p}$ bilat. UE PNF exercises.

   Translation:
   _____
   _____
   _____
   _____

5. In chart:
   Dx: MS; R/O OBS.

   Translation:
   _____
   _____
   _____

6. In PT note:
   The patient is a below the knee amputee with a patellar tendon bearing prosthesis with a solid ankle cushion heel foot.

   Translation:
   _____
   _____
   _____

7. In OT note:
   The patient's heart rate increased 20 beats per minute after only 2 minutes of self-care activities of daily living.

   Translation:
   _____
   _____
   _____

8. In PT note:
   The patient ambulated in the parallel bars full weight bearing left lower extremity for approximately 20 feet twice with minimal assistance of 1 person.

   Translation:
   _____
   _____
   _____

22

9. In OT or PT note:
   Upper extremity strength is normal throughout bilaterally.

   Translation:

   _____

   _____

10. In PT or OT note:
    Short Term Goal: decrease dependence in transfers wheelchair to bed to moderate assistance within one week.

    Translation:

    _____

    _____

Answers to "Using Abbreviations: Worksheet 1" are included in Appendix A.

Using Abbreviations: WORKSHEET 2

Translate each phrase or sentence written with abbreviations into full English phrases or sentences. Translate each sentence or phrase written in English into a sentence or phrase written with abbreviations.

1. Pt. c/o Ⓡ hip pain p̄ amb ~ 300 ft. × 1 c̄ a walker FWB Ⓡ LE.

   Translation:

   _____

   _____

   _____

   _____

   _____

   _____

   _____

   _____

2. You must write in the chart: The patient may be 50 percent partial weight bearing left lower extremity per verbal order of Dr. Smith.

   Translation:

   _____

   _____

   _____

3. Order written in chart: D/C US in area of Ⓡ SI joint.

   Translation:

   _____

   _____

   _____

4. D̲x̲: Fx Ⓛ clavicle & subluxation Ⓛ SC joint.

   Translation:

   _____

   _____

   _____

   _____

5. In physician's note: FBS upon adm was over 300.

   Translation:

   _____

   _____

   _____

6. D̲i̲a̲g̲n̲o̲s̲i̲s̲: left cerebrovascular accident.

   Translation:

   _____

7. Muscle function test reveals good strength throughout the upper extremities bilaterally.

   Translation:

   _____

   _____

   _____

24

8. X-ray reveals fracture of the left third metacarpal immediately proximal to the metacarpalphalangeal joint.

Translation:

_____

_____

_____

9. Order for you to write in the chart: To occupational therapy for activities of daily living per verbal order of Dr. Jones

Translation:

_____

_____

10. In the physician's note: <u>Imp</u>: peripheral neuropathy; R/O CNS dysfunction.

Translation:

_____

_____

_____

_____

_____

_____

_____

_____

Answers to "Using Abbreviations: Worksheet 2" are provided in Appendix A.

Medical Terminology 4

Before any healthcare professional can begin reading or writing SOAP notes in an acceptable manner, she or he must be familiar with the terminology commonly used in medical writing. Most of the terms have Latin-based prefixes, suffixes, or roots. It is often easy to ascertain the meaning of a particular term if the more commonly used prefixes, suffixes, and roots are known.

term = prefix + *root*   *Example:* Sclero*derma*

                 or

term = *root* + suffix   *Example:* Osteoporosis

                 or

term = prefix + *root* + suffix   *Example:* Syn*dactyl*ism

Learning medical terminology, its prefixes, suffixes, and roots, is outside the scope of this workbook. Some basic knowledge of medical terminology is assumed.

The following worksheets should serve as a review of medical terminology. The terms used in these worksheets are encountered frequently by therapists and assistants. If you are unfamiliar with the terms and definitions used in these worksheets, it is suggested that you review medical terminology before continuing in this workbook. The list of references in Appendix E of this book should prove helpful to you in reviewing medical terminology, if needed.

Medical Terminology: WORKSHEET 1

Part I. Write the appropriate term for the definition.

1. Tumor of the bone _____

2. Abnormally low blood sugar _____

3. Beneath the skin _____

4. Above the symphysis pubis _____

5. Pertaining to the back of the body _____

6. Toward the head _____

7. Abnormal redness of the skin _____

8. Between the ribs _____

9. Front of the body _____ or _____

10. Conducting toward a structure _____

Part II. Write the appropriate definition for the term listed.

1. Symphysis pubis _____

_____

2. Cardiomegaly _____

_____

3. Menisectomy _____

_____

4. Chondroma _____

_____

5. Arthrodesis _____

_____

6. Craniotomy _____

_____

7. Neurology _____

_____

8. Anesthesia _____

_____

9. Phlebitis _____

_____

10. Hypertension _____

_____

Answers to "Medical Terminology: Worksheet 1" are provided in Appendix A.

Medical Terminology: WORKSHEET 2

Part I. Write the appropriate term for the definition.

1. Joint inflammation _____

2. Inspection of joint with a scope _____

3. Disease of a muscle _____

4. Difficult or bad breathing _____

5. Lack of coordination _____

6. Softening of cartilage _____

7. Inflammation of the brain _____

8. Tumor of the meninges _____

9. Paralysis of one half of the body _____

10. Beneath the clavicle _____

Part II. Write the appropriate definition for the term listed.

1. Analgesia _____

2. Bilateral _____

3. Contralateral _____

4. Aphasia _____

5. Tendinitis _____

6. Bradykinesia _____

7. Dysphagia _____

8. Arthralgia _____

9. Cerebromalacia _____

10. Costochondral _____

Answers to "Medical Terminology: Worksheet 2" are provided in Appendix A.

5 Stating the Problem

In many facilities, the major problem or problems that have brought the patient to you for treatment are stated before actually beginning the SOAP note itself. This is usually stated as *Problem:* or *Dx:*. The *Problem* part of the note can be stated as the patient's chief complaint, the diagnosis, or a loss of function. It may be medical, psychological, or functional.

In some facilities the pertinent history or medical information taken from the chart is included in the *problem* area. In others it is the first information written in the O part of the note. For the purposes of this workbook, you are expected to state this information in the *problem* area of the note, since it is not the result of tests you have conducted (your interview or measurements). Included would be information such as the following:

- **Past surgeries** affecting the present condition/treatment (example: hx of Ⓡ total knee replacement in 1992).
- **Past conditions/diseases** affecting the present condition/treatment (example: hx of Ⓡ CVA in 1990).
- **Present conditions/diseases** affecting the present condition/treatment (example: hypertension, CHF).
- **Test results** affecting the present condition/treatment (example: x-ray reveals fx Ⓡ tibial plateau).
- **Recent or past surgery** affecting present condition/treatment (example: Ⓛ total hip replacement performed on [date]).

Two examples of the problem part of the note are as follows:

1. Dx: Ⓛ hemiplegia resulting from craniotomy for removal of tumor on 9-12-94.
2. 58 yr. old ♂ c̄ Ⓛ BK amputation on 7-17-93 2° PVD. Hx of diabetes.

There are no worksheets on writing the problem. As you practice writing notes on the worksheets that follow, you are expected to state the problem (if it is given to you) before you write the rest of the note. You will get much practice at stating the problem in completing this workbook.

Writing **6**
Subjective (*S*)

The subjective part of the note is the section in which the therapist is able to state the information received from the patient that is relevant to the patient's present condition. Subjective information is necessary to plan the objective assessment of the patient and to justify or explain certain goals that are set with the patient. For example, third-party payers, utilization review auditors, and quality assurance auditors may question assessing a patient on 16 steps or teaching a patient to go up and down a flight of 16 steps (and why it is taking the patient longer than other patients his age to become independent) unless the subjective part of the note includes documentation that the patient has 16 steps to enter his home.

Categorizing Items as Subjective

An item belongs under subjective if

- *The patient* (or significant other) tells the therapist or assistant of activities that the patient can no longer perform due to the patient's current condition. This is often referred to as **prior level of function.**
- *The patient* (or significant other) tells the therapist or assistant the patient's history.
- *The patient* (or significant other) tells the therapist or assistant something about the patient's **lifestyle** or **home situation.**
- *The patient* tells the therapist or assistant his or her **emotions** or **attitudes** (Example: ''I'm really angry about . . .).
- *The patient* states his or her **goals** (or the significant other states his or her goals for the patient).
- *The patient* voices a **complaint.**
- *The patient* reports a **response to treatment** (Example: a decrease in pain intensity).
- It is **anything** *the patient* (or a designated significant other) tells the therapist or assistant that is **relevant to the patient's case or present condition.**

The relevant history obtained from the chart may be stated under the problem (in some facilities, it is stated under *O*, Objective). It does not belong under Subjective because *it is not something that the patient (or significant other) told the therapist directly.*

The Use of "Patient"

Generally, the *S* section of the note should be as brief (yet complete) as possible. It is acceptable to use "Pt." the first time, but do not repeat it with every sentence. It is assumed, unless otherwise stated, that the information in this section came from the patient.

EXAMPLE

Incorrect: Pt. c/o pain in Ⓡ low back area. Pt. states pain ↓'s c̄ rest. Pt. states is unable to work or perform most ADLs because pt. cannot sit >5 min. 2° pain.

This Is a Waste of Time and Space!

Correct: Pt. c/o pain in Ⓡ low back area. States pain ↓'s c̄ rest; is unable to work or perform most ADLs because cannot sit >5 min. 2° pain.

Abbreviations and Medical Terminology

Appropriate abbreviations and use of medical terminology are expected. Correct spelling is necessary for the therapist to be represented appropriately as a professional. The most concise (yet complete) wording should be used. Full sentences are not necessary if the idea is complete (this varies from facility to facility).

EXAMPLE

WORDY
The pt. states pain began ~3 wks. ago Wed.

MORE CONCISE
Pt. states onset of pain on (date).

Organization

It is important for the sake of the other professionals reading the note to organize the note by topic. Often, subcategories, or headings, such as *prior level of function, c/o (some facilities use functional c/o to emphasize the importance of the c/o to the patient's function), home situation, Pt. goals, lifestyle, hx, pain behavior,* are used. To which of the two examples below would you rather refer if you were looking for particular information?

EXAMPLE

1. Pt. c/o pain Ⓡ ankle when Ⓡ ankle is in a dependent position. Lives alone & must prepare all meals. Pt.'s goal is to play basketball again. Denies previous use of crutches. Denies any other pain or dizziness. Describes 3 steps s̄ a handrail at entrance to his home. States hx of a fall at home & feeling his ankle "pop." States played basketball 3x/wk. PTA.

2. C/o: pain Ⓡ ankle when Ⓡ ankle is in a dependent position. Denies any other pain or dizziness. Hx: States fell at home & felt his Ⓡ ankle "pop." Denies use of crutches PTA. Home situation: Describes 3 steps s̄ handrail at the entrance to his home. States lives alone & must prepare all meals. Prior level of function/Pt. goals: States played basketball 3x/wk. PTA; pt.'s goal is to play basketball again.

In the first example, getting a clear picture of the patient's status is difficult. The second example is much easier to read.

Almost every note should include information on patient's *c/o, prior level of function, goals,* and view of his or her own functioning prior to admission. Many should also include the *home situation,* because this section describes the physical arrangement of the home and the significant other(s) available to support or assist the patient in functioning or complying with therapy at home.

Do not include information or subcategories in the *S* section of the note just for the sake of inclusion. The purpose of information included in any part of the note is to address the patient's present condition and problems accurately and to assist in monitoring progress, revising the patient's program, and/or discontinuing therapy when necessary. Information that is not relevant to the patient's present condition, level of functioning, or need for function at home should not be included. Irrelevant information wastes time, makes the note unnecessarily long, and may confuse all those who read the chart for purposes of case management, quality care assessment, discharge planning, utilization review, or reimbursement. For further information on reimbursement issues, see Appendix D.

Verbs

S statements frequently contain a verb which indicates that the statement is subjective and not taken from the chart. Verbs frequently used are *states, describes, denies, indicates, c/o.*

Quoting the Patient Verbatim

At times, quoting the patient verbatim is the most appropriate method of conveying subjective information. Some reasons for using direct quotes from the patient or a family member might be

- To illustrate **confusion** or **loss of memory.** (Example: Pt. frequently states, "My mother will make everything all right. I want my mother." The patient is 80 years old.)
- To illustrate **denial.** (Example: Pt. states, "I don't need home health PT. I'll be fine once I'm in my own home." The patient is dependent in amb & lives alone.)
- To illustrate a patient's **attitude toward therapy.** (Example: Pt. stated, "I don't think any therapy can get rid of my pain.")
- To illustrate the patient's **use of abusive language.** (Example: Pt. stated to therapist, "Keep your __ hands off of me.")

Using Information Taken from a Family Member

Information taken from an interview with a patient's family member can be included in the following manner:

Dx: Ⓛ CVA c̄ Ⓡ hemiparesis & aphasia.
S: (All of the following information was taken from pt.'s daughter. Pt. is unable to verbalize 2° aphasia.) H̲x̲: Pt. amb indep PTA. H̲ome situation̲: Pt. lives c̄ daughter & daughter's husband in a 1-story home c̄ 3 steps c̄ handrail Ⓛ ascending to enter the home. Home has carpeted & linoleum surfaces s̄ throw rugs. Pt.'s bedroom is ~7 ft. from the bathroom & ~15 ft. from the kitchen or living room. Daughter works full time. F̲amily goals̲: Pt. must be able to stay alone during the day while daughter works.

Examples of use of a combination of information taken from the patient and a family member follow in corresponding PT & OT notes regarding the same patient:

Dx: Peripheral neuropathy bilat. LEs; COPD. H̲x̲: Htn, ASHD.
S: C̲/o̲: Pt. c/o SOB ā assessment; immediately p̄ assessment, indicated that SOB had ↑; 5 min. p̄ exercise, stated SOB had ↓. H̲x̲: Pt.'s husband stated pt. hx of COPD for 10 yrs.

Prior level of function: Pt. has not amb for the past 2 mo. & has required assist. for transfers 2° SOB & weakness. Husband stated Pt. transferred & amb s̄ assist. device indep prior to past 2 mo. Home situation: Husband described a 1-story home; a ramp is present to access the entrance to the home. All floor surfaces are linoleum. Furthest distance pt. must amb is ~50 ft. Husband is home full time to care for Pt. Pt. goals: Both stated long term goal of Pt. amb indep, c̄ or s̄ assist. device, & short term goal of indep transfers.

Dx: Peripheral neuropathy bilat. LEs; COPD. Hx: Htn, ASHD.

S: C/o: Pt. stated she cannot tolerate both PT & OT bid 2° fatigue. Husband states Pt. has needed assist. for dressing LEs, transfers w/c ↔ toilet & has required set-up for a sponge bath with assist. in bathing LEs. Hx: Pt. states 10 yr. hx of COPD. LE weakness began ~2 mo. ago. Prior level of function: Husband states Pt. was able to handle all self-care activities until 2 mo. ago. Pt. goals: Both stated functional goal of indep transfers w/c ↔ toilet, indep in bathing & dressing, & Pt. would like to be able to bathe in the tub or shower. Home situation: Husband is home full time to care for Pt. but states he is having back pain after transferring the Pt.

Writing Subjective Information in Functional Outcomes Reporting

Functional outcomes reporting is a style of note writing that focuses on the patient's function. This style of note writing can use the SOAP format as well as other formats. When using a SOAP format and functional outcomes reporting in combination, the Subjective portion of the note should focus on the patient's function, specifically what the patient cannot do at home because of his or her physical impairments. Headings frequently used would be *prior level of function, current level of function, home situation,* and *patient goals.* The subjective information used in a functional outcomes environment can be used later as a guide to whether the patient is improving in function.

Writing Interim (Progress) Notes

The *S* portion of the note is optional in an interim note. It is used if there is an update of previous information or if there is relevant new information to convey. Listing information that reflects a temporary mood of discouragement in the patient is not necessary and could confuse those reading the note. Of course, irrelevant information is never appropriate.

Subjective information addressed in previously set goals for the patient should be addressed in the interim note. For example, if the patient initially stated that his or her pain prevented the performance of functional activities and rated his or her level of pain using a pain scale, and the therapist and patient set a goal for decreasing the patient's pain by three levels on the pain scale in one week, the patient's functional level and level of pain should be addressed in the interim note at the end of the week. Although information such as pain level is subjective, it can be a method of showing progress when combined with functional progress.

A patient's subjective **response to treatment**—such as pain following exercise, pain felt with movement, a decrease in pain after treatment, or fatigue after exercise—can be reported in an interim note. This information can be used to document improvement and reinforce objective measurements. For example, if a patient used to feel pain with exercise or a certain movement, such as bending forward or backward, and no longer feels pain, then the patient has improved in pain-free mobility, making him or her more functional in ADL.

Another type of subjective information that can be addressed in the interim note is information regarding the **patient's compliance and/or other health conditions during the week.** After interviewing the patient, the therapist can document whether the patient is doing prescribed exercises at home and how often. (Example: Pt. states she is performing her exercises in the a.m. and late night time but performs exercises at midday ~50% of the time.) Medical problems, such as cold or flu, that could help explain why a patient did not progress during a week or two of therapy can be documented.

The patient's **level of functioning at home** is still another area that can be addressed in the subjective section of the note. Unless the therapist is employed by a home health agency, she or he must rely on the patient to convey information about function at home. A patient may appear to be making only minimal progress in therapy on impairments of ROM or strength (objective measures of the degree of impairment) but may be making large improvements in functional ability at home. Thus, subjective information regarding functional activities at home should be included in the interim notes.

Writing Discharge Notes

The completeness of the S section of a discharge note varies greatly from facility to facility. In some facilities, the discharge note is similar to an interim note and only updates the patient's status since the most recent interim note was written. In other facilities, the S portion of the discharge note more completely summarizes the patient's complaints and home situation, as well as whether the patient believes the goals set were achieved and whether the patient feels ready to function at home. For the purposes of this workbook, the discharge note is to be considered a complete summary of the patient's status upon discharge from therapy, and all of the relevant subjective information regarding the patient should be addressed.

Summary

The S portion of the note should include relevant information that will assist the therapist with setting goals for the patient, planning the patient's treatment, and deciding when to discontinue treatment. Irrelevant information should not be included, but care needs to be taken to address the patient's situation and level of functioning at home, both at the present time and prior to the onset of the patient's current problem.

The worksheets that follow will give you practice in the skills needed to write the S part of a note. Also included are some exercises in stating the problem. After reviewing Chapter 5, "Stating the Problem," and the material in this chapter, working with the following worksheets, and using the answer sheets to correct the worksheets, you should be able to easily write the problem and subjective portions of a note.

Writing Subjective (S): WORKSHEET 1 (Also Included: Stating the Problem)

Part I. Mark the statements that should be placed in the S category by placing an S on the line before the statement. Also mark the information that belongs in the Problem portion of the note by writing Prob. on the line before the statement.

1. _____ Pt. c/o pain Ⓛ wrist.

2. _____ Pt. will demonstrate a normal gait pattern 95% of the time within 3 wks.

3. _____ Flexion in lying reproduces pt.'s worst Ⓡ LE pain.

4. _____ Pulsed US @ 1.5–2.0 W/cm² to Ⓡ upper trapezius for 5 min.

5. _____ Strength: N throughout all extremities.

6. _____ States hx of COPD since 1990.

7. _____ Pt. has good rehab potential.

8. _____ Will be seen by OT 3×/wk. as an O.P.

9. _____ States onset of pain was in July 1994.

10. _____ Hx: CA of the colon c̄ colostomy in 1993.

11. _____ AROM: WNL bilat LEs.

12. _____ Pt. has been referred to home health services for further PT & OT.

13. _____ ↑ AROM Ⓡ shoulder to WNL within 2 mo.

14. _____ Denies pain c̄ cough.

15. _____ Will initiate OT post-op per TKR pathway protocol.

16. _____ Hx: Htn, ASHD, CAD.

17. _____ Pt. was unable to communicate verbally & did not follow commands well; thus, objective eval. was limited.

18. _____ Indep in donning/doffing prosthesis within 1 wk.

19. _____ Gait: Independent c̄ crutches 10% PWB Ⓡ LE for 150 ft. × 2.

20. _____ C/o pain Ⓛ low back p̄ sitting for ~10 min.

21. _____ Will inquire if pt. can be referred to OT & speech therapy.

22. _____ States his goal is to return to work ASAP.

Part II. The following is information regarding several patients' diagnoses and chief complaints. This information was taken from the chart or received from the physician's office. Write the information listed in each case into the Problem portion of a note.

1. The patient is an outpatient & the patient's diagnosis received from the physician is "right shoulder bursitis."

   Correct statement: _____

2. The patient had a right cerebrovascular accident approximately 1 year ago with residual left hemiparesis. He now comes to you as an outpatient. The patient's present diagnosis from the physician is "left shoulder subluxation."

   Correct statement: _____

_____

3. The patient is an inpatient with a diagnosis of respiratory failure. She has a history of chronic obstructive pulmonary disease and congestive heart failure.

Correct statement: _____

Part III. Below you will find the familiar headings discussed for the *S* portion of a note. Each is followed by five blanks (more than are needed for the exercise). Below these headings are nine statements to be included in the note. Write the number of each in the blank following its appropriate heading. The statements you list following each heading should be in the order in which they would logically appear in a note (for instance, 1–5–3 might make more sense than if you were to order them 3–1–5). You may wish to write the note out on a separate piece of paper to assist yourself with this task.

       A. c/o: _____, _____, _____, _____, _____

       B. Pt. goals: _____, _____, _____, _____, _____

       C. Home situation: _____, _____, _____, _____, _____

       D. Prior level of function: _____, _____, _____, _____, _____

       E. Hx: _____, _____, _____, _____, _____

1. Pt. c/o ℞ shoulder pain "all over the shoulder."
2. States fell at home & landed on a step on ℞ shoulder.
3. States lives alone at home & drives herself to therapy.
4. Describes pain as constant $\bar{c}$ intensity of 6 (0 = no pain, 10 = worst possible pain).
5. C/o difficulty lifting heavy cooking pots & closing zippers on the back of her clothing.
6. States pain ↓'s $\bar{c}$ rest & is at its worst while Pt. is at work.
7. States she wants to be able to close her zippers & cook $\bar{s}$ assist. upon completion of therapy.
8. Denies previous shoulder pain/stiffness/inflammation.
9. States was able to fasten all clothing & was completely independent with all cooking activities and activities of daily living prior to her fall at home.

Part IV. Rewrite the following *S* statements in a more clear, concise, and professional manner. Also, list the heading under which the statement should be placed.

1. States she had a fall in her living room. (Question: What information from the patient would make this statement more informative and useful?)

    a. Heading: _____

    b. Corrected statement: _____

    c. Answer to question: _____

    _____

2. States pain began around 5:00 p.m. a wk. ago Wed.

    a. Heading: _____

    b. Corrected statement: _____

3. States she is kind of sore today in her ℞ foot. (Question: What information from the Pt. would make this statement more informative and useful?)

    a. Heading: _____

    b. Corrected statement: _____

    c. Answer to question: _____

    _____

4. States she lives alone. States she has two steps to enter her home. States the steps have a handrail which is on the right when a person is going up the stairs.

   a. <u>Heading:</u> _____

   b. <u>Corrected statement:</u> _____

   _____

   _____

5. States the pain goes from her right hand up her right forearm today. The pain is allowing her to type for only five minutes at a time.

   a. <u>Heading:</u> _____

   b. <u>Corrected statement:</u> _____

   _____

Part V. The following are the notes to yourself that you jotted down while reading the chart and talking with two patients. The first information is from an initial assessment; the second information is from a follow-up, or interim, assessment. (While taking notes for yourself, you did not consult Hospital XYZ's approved abbreviations list.)

From the Chart

58 yr. old, male
minor ligamentous injury Ⓡ knee

From the Pt.

Ⓡ Knee pain—constant, "burning"—7 on 0–10 scale
↓ Pain c̄ rest
↑ Pain c̄ walking
No pain bending Ⓡ knee
No using crutches before
Lives c̄ wife—apartment on 2nd floor—no elevator—9 steps to enter c̄ handrail on the Ⓛ going ↑
Fell at work—landing on Ⓡ knee 1st
Wants to be able to access apt. independently (short term)
Wants to be able to resume former busy lifestyle, including returning to work as soon as poss.
   (long term)
Occupation—carpenter

1. Write the above information into the Problem and *S* portions of a note. Your partial note should be written to be an acceptable part of the patient's medical record at Hospital XYZ (using approved abbreviations).

   _____

   _____

   _____

   _____

   _____

   _____

_____

_____

_____

_____

From the Chart

This is an interim note on an outpatient. You have received no new information from the patient's physician. For your information: the patient's diagnosis is minor ligamentous injury Ⓛ wrist. The patient is a 33-year-old male.

From the Patient

Ⓛ hand & wrist are puffy & feel stiff when the patient tries to move them
puffiness worse after work
types at work—up to 8 hrs. a day—MD told him to limit typing to 4 hrs. a day until stops swelling
pain w/ typing—5 on a 0–10 scale
↓ pain w/ rest
↑ pain w/ grasping or wt. bearing activities Ⓛ UE
no use of splint before
lives w/ wife—no previous injuries
won't have to cook or lift heavy objects at home until ready
fell at work—landed on Ⓛ hand w/ wrist extended
wants to be able to hold a fork w/o pain (short term)—trouble eating w/ Ⓡ hand—Ⓛ hand
    dominant
wants to be able to return to former busy lifestyle—includes typing at work (long term)
occupation—transcriptionist

2. Write the above information into the *S* portion of the note. Your partial note should be written to be an acceptable part of the patient's medical record at Hospital XYZ (using approved abbreviations).

_____

_____

_____

_____

_____

_____

_____

_____

_____

_____

_____

_____

Answers to "Writing Subjective (S): Worksheet 1" are provided in Appendix A.

Writing Subjective (S): WORKSHEET 2 (Also Included: Stating the Problem)

Part I. Below you will find the familiar headings discussed for the *S* portion of a note. Each is followed by five blanks (more than are needed for the exercise). Below these headings are nine statements to be included in the note. Write the number of each in the blank following its appropriate heading. The statements you list after each heading should be in the order in which they would logically appear in a note (for instance, 1–5–3 may make more sense than if you were to order them 3–1–5). You may wish to write the note out on a separate piece of paper to assist yourself with this task.

    A. Present c/o: _____, _____, _____, _____, _____

    B. Hx: _____, _____, _____, _____, _____

    C. Home situation: _____, _____, _____, _____, _____

    D. Goals: _____, _____, _____, _____, _____

    E. Prior level of function: _____, _____, _____, _____, _____

1. States fell @ home & fx Ⓛ hip.
2. States needs to be able to amb c̄ walker indep ~15 ft. in order to return home c̄ her husband.
3. States lives c̄ husband in her own home; husband is home all day.
4. Describes 3 steps c̄ a handrail Ⓛ ascending at entrance of her home.
5. States has "bad heart trouble" but denies pain or difficulty presently.
6. States used a walker since 1988 when she fx Ⓡ hip.
7. States is hard of hearing.
8. Pt. c/o pain Ⓛ hip c̄ standing NWB Ⓛ LE.
9. States would like to return home c̄ her husband p̄ D/C.

Part II. Rewrite the following *S* statements in a more clear, concise, and professional manner. Also, list the heading under which the statement should be placed.

1. Pain is in her right leg down to, but not including, the knee. (Question: What other information regarding the patient's pain would help this statement to be more useful and informative?)

    a. Heading: _____

    b. Corrected statement: _____

    _____

    c. Answer to question: _____

    _____

    _____

2. States he depended on his wife to give him a bath before this stroke & he plans to continue to depend on her to give him a bath now.

    a. Heading: _____

    b. Corrected statement: _____

    _____

3. Complains of not being able to put on her clothes by herself.

    a. Heading: _____

    b. Corrected statement: _____

4. Says she never used a walker before this present adm to Hospital XYZ.

    a. <u>Heading</u>: _____

    b. <u>Corrected statement</u>: _____

    _____

Part III. Mark the statements that should be placed in the *S* category by placing an *S* on the line before the statement. Also mark the information that belongs in the Problem portion of the note by writing Prob. on the line before the statement.

1. _____ Will request an order for OT to assist $\bar{c}$ dressing.

2. _____ DTRs 2+ throughout LEs except 3+ ⓡ KJ.

3. _____ Amb training, beginning // bars & progressing to a walker.

4. _____ States was in a car accident & Pt.'s car was hit broadside on the passenger side.

5. _____ <u>Goal</u>: Indep walker amb 150 ft. × 2 FWB within 2 wks.

6. _____ Eval. not complete because Pt. does not follow commands consistently.

7. _____ C/o inability to zip her dresses behind her back.

8. _____ <u>Transfers</u>: Supine ↔ sit $\bar{c}$ min +1 assist.

9. _____ <u>Proprioception</u>: ↓ noted throughout entire ⓡ UE.

10. _____ <u>Hx</u>: TIA in 1989, ASHD, CHF.

11. _____ C/o pain in "entire" Ⓛ LE $\bar{c}$ active or passive movement of the knee.

12. _____ AROM Ⓛ knee to 0–90° within 2 wks.

13. _____ BID @ B/S:

14. _____ Pt. will demonstrate knowledge of proper back care & ADL by discussion of ADL $\bar{c}$ therapist & through 90% correct performance on an obstacle course in back care & ADL.

15. _____ C/o itching in scar Ⓛ wrist ~2×/hr.

16. _____ Will request an order for PT for assessment of gross motor functioning.

17. _____ <u>Sensation</u>: Absent to light touch & pin prick throughout L5 distribution.

18. _____ Pt. will be given written & verbal instruction in home exercise & walking program (attached).

19. _____ States would like to return to his daughter's house until he no longer needs the walker.

Part IV. The following are the notes to yourself that you jotted down while reading the chart and talking with your patient. (While taking notes for yourself, you did not consult Hospital XYZ's approved abbreviations list.)

From the Chart

Diagnosis is contusion left hip

From the Pt.

Ⓛ hip pain when FWB Ⓛ LE—8 on a 0–10 scale
Total hip replacement Ⓛ 1990—used walker then
no hip pain sitting or supine
Apartment with elevator—lives alone—curbs only
fell in kitchen on Ⓛ hip in a.m.—able to get up s̄ help—pain throughout day—went to ER late
    p.m.
did not use an assistive device before his injury and walked independently
did all ADL tasks independently prior to his injury
eventually would like to independently perform all ADL tasks s̄ walker
currently spends time in a wheelchair rented by the family

1. Write the above information into the Problem and *S* portions of a note. Your partial note should
be written to be an acceptable part of the patient's medical record at Hospital XYZ (using
approved abbreviations).

_____

_____

_____

_____

_____

_____

_____

_____

_____

_____

Answers to "Writing Subjective (S): Worksheet 2" are provided in Appendix A.

7 Writing Objective (O)

The objective part of the note is the section in which the results of measurements performed and the therapist's objective observations of the patient are recorded. Objective data are the *measurable* or *observable* information used to plan patient treatment. The testing procedures that produce objective data are *repeatable*. Objective information written in one note can be compared with measurements taken and recorded in the past. It will also serve as comparative data in the future, as the patient's progress is monitored and reassessed.

Categorizing Items into Objective

An item belongs under objective if

- It is part of the patient's **history** taken **from the medical record and relevant to the current problem.** Note: Only certain facilities include information from the medical record under *O*.

EXAMPLE

> **O:** Hx: ASHD, CHF, COPD. S/P fx Ⓛ hip c̄ prosthesis insertion 1 yr.

- It is a **result of the therapist's objective measurements or observations** (must be measurable and reproducible data; may use data base, flow sheets, or charts and summarize data here).

EXAMPLE

> **O:** AROM: WNL throughout UEs & LEs except 120° Ⓛ shoulder flexion noted.

- It is **part of the treatment** given to a patient (particularly modifications used, number of repetitions tolerated, pain relieved or caused). This documentation provides information to anyone who might treat the patient as to what was done in therapy on a certain date. It is also done to inform both those reimbursing the treatment and those who might read the medical record as a legal document of what specifically was done with the patient.

EXAMPLE

> **O:** Treatment given this date: Mobilization to Ⓡ shoulder (inferior glides, long axis distraction), AROM & PROM exercises, 10 reps x 3 each isometric exercises for shoulder medial & lateral rotators, & ice massage.

- **Patient education** activities (particularly specific exercises taught to the patient). Note: Many agencies accrediting patient care facilities are very interested in written evidence of what we teach our patients and their families.

EXAMPLE

> **O:** Patient Education: Received instruction in home exercise program & was indep in same program (attached).

As mentioned previously, facilities differ widely as to where and how much pertinent information from the medical record becomes part of the therapy note as well as *if* it is included. Some therapists believe that if the information is relevant enough to state, it should go with the diagnosis when the patient's problem is stated. Other facilities have the policy that information from the patient's medical record should be included in the objective section of the note because it is information that the therapist did not obtain from the patient directly (and therefore is *not* subjective) and the section including the diagnosis is extremely brief. Still other facilities do not include information from the medical record under *O* since it is *not* a result of direct testing performed by the therapist. Upon arriving at a facility to practice, the best policy for students to follow is to enquire as to which style of note writing is used. For the purposes of this workbook, you will be expected to briefly include information from the medical record after the diagnosis or chief complaint when you initially state the patient's problem.

Abbreviations and Medical Terminology

Appropriate use of abbreviations and medical terminology is expected, as well as correct spelling.

The following pages discuss some methods of recording objective data. Use them as a reference. Clarity and conciseness are important.

Organization

Information should be organized, easy to read, and easy to find.

EXAMPLE

> POORLY WRITTEN
> **O:** Strength is N throughout UEs. ROM is WNL throughout UEs. Ⓡ toes are warm to touch and coloration is normal. Ⓛ LE AROM is WNL throughout. Ⓡ LE strength & ROM not assessed due to long leg cast. Ⓛ LE strength is N throughout. Able to manage NWB status Ⓛ LE indep.
>
> PROPERLY WRITTEN
> **O:** UEs & Ⓛ LE: Strength & AROM are WNL throughout. Ⓡ LE: Strength & AROM not assessed due to long leg cast. Toes warm to touch & coloration WNL. Able to manage NWB status indep.

Categories

In order to organize objective data better and make it easy to read, objective information is divided into categories or headings. The headings or categories used depend on the patient's deficits and diagnosis.

Headings or categories can be based on the *types of tests and measurements performed*. This type of organization is helpful when the patient has deficits in several parts of the body or some type of generalized problem. Examples of categories include the following:

Ambulation
Transfers
Balance
ROM
Strength
Sensation

Headings or categories can also be based on *areas of the body and functional skills*. Use of this type of organization is found when many of the patient's deficits are located in one or two parts of the body. Examples of categories include the following:

Ambulation
ADL
UEs
LEs
Trunk

Or

Ambulation
ADL
Ⓡ Extremities
Ⓛ Extremities
Trunk

Placement of Objective Data into Categories

Placing objective data into categories depends on the diagnosis and deficits of the individual patient.

EXAMPLES

1. For the physical therapist, a patient with a low back problem may show deficits in the areas of gait, many aspects of the trunk, and the lower extremities as well as body mechanics during transfers and activities of daily living. The information would be divided into categories that would list the information regarding the trunk, lower extremities, and gait separately: gait, ADL, trunk, LEs, UEs. For the occupational therapist, the patient may show deficits in lifting abilities needed in her or his work, body mechanics, and daily self-care activities. The information would be divided into categories listing the deficit areas separately: vocational activities, body mechanics, self-care activities.

2. A patient with a diagnosis of left cerebrovascular accident might show deficits in many aspects regarding the right side of the body including decreased active moment, a change in tone, decreased sensation, changed deep tendon reflexes, decreased coordination, decreased fine motor abilities. In order to make the information clearer and the deficits easier to read, the information regarding the right

extremities should be separated from that for the left extremities because the left extremities are essentially normal. The trunk is one entity and should not be divided into different categories. Gait deviations and deficits in dressing and grooming exist and should each be described in a separate category. Deficits are found in other functional activities such as transfers and rolling. These functional activities can be listed under the categories of transfers & bed mobility. The categories used by the physical therapist might be gait, transfers, bed mobility, Ⓡ extremities, Ⓛ extremities, trunk. The categories used by the occupational therapist might be transfers, bed mobility, dressing, grooming, Ⓡ extremities, Ⓛ extremities.

3. A patient with colon cancer might show many deficits in strength and range of motion. These deficits occur in all of the extremities when the physical therapist assesses the patient. Transfers and ambulation need work. The patient's endurance is low. For the physical therapist, the information might best be divided according to the patient's basic areas of deficit: ambulation, transfers, strength, AROMs, endurance. When the occupational therapist assesses this patient, the patient also shows deficits in UE strength and AROM as well as deficits in endurance, feeding, grooming, and dressing activities. For the occupational therapist, the information might also best be divided according to areas of deficit: feeding, grooming, dressing, UE strength, UE AROMs, endurance.

4. When the therapist assesses a young pediatric patient, the assessment reveals low muscle tone, normal ROM, deficits in strength and stability, a delay in righting reactions, and deficits in mobility. These areas can all be listed under the category of gross motor skills. The child shows appropriate fine motor skills and deficient sensory functioning as well as difficulties in feeding. The therapist chooses to divide the categories into ADL, gross motor, fine motor, and sensory.

Use of categories also varies from one clinical facility to another. Certain facilities require therapists to categorize information on all patients in the same manner despite differences in diagnoses and deficits between patients. (For example, all notes in one facility might have the categories *gait, ADL, strength, ROM, sensation.*) Other facilities give the therapists more freedom to categorize information in the manner they deem most efficient and organized. For the purposes of this workbook, you will be expected to choose the most appropriate categories for each patient's specific diagnosis and deficits.

Within the objective portion of a note, the categories can be arranged using a number of different methods. Some clinicians list the functional activities (gait, transfers, ADL) first because they believe that functional activities are the most important. Others believe that the extremities and trunk or tests performed should be listed first because the information on ROM, strength, and so forth, is needed to understand the reasons for the deficits in function. Most of the audiences for SOAP notes (physicians, insurance reviewers, lawyers, utilization reviewers, social workers) prefer listing the functional activities first, with the reasons for the deficits in function listed after the functional deficits. For the purposes of this workbook, you are expected to address functional activities before listing the extremities or specific tests performed.

Within any individual category in the objective section of a note, the information is organized in the most logical order possible. Usually one joint at a time is described, and joints are addressed from proximal to distal. Information is otherwise grouped as efficiently as possible within this framework.

EXAMPLE

<u>UEs</u>: AROM: WNL except for 80° Ⓡ shoulder flexion & 90° elbow flexion. STRENGTH: G− throughout shoulder musculature, G+ biceps, G triceps, F in musculature controlling the wrist & fingers. SENSATION: Intact throughout.

Methods of Recording Objective Data

In many facilities, complete sentences are not necessary, but information should be clear enough to get the idea across.

EXAMPLE

UNCLEAR
AROM: Ⓛ ankle in cast.

CLEAR
AROM: Ⓛ ankle not assessed due to short leg cast Ⓛ LE.

At times, using a chart gets the information across in the most complete manner.

EXAMPLE (Correct Method)

AROM: Ⓛ finger & thumb extension/flexion is as follows:

Digit	MCP	PIP	DIP
1	20–0–45°	10–0–20°	
2	10–0–40°	0–15°	0–2°
3	10–0–40°	0–30°	10–0–5°
4	10–0–38°	0–10°	0–8°
5	20–0–47°	0–5°	0–5°

Sometimes, a standard ROM or muscle testing chart, flow sheet, or some other standardized chart can be used (many therapy departments have these available for use). Instead of giving detailed information within the note, the therapist can refer to the flow sheet or chart and attach a copy to the note.

EXAMPLE

AROM Ⓡ UE: See attached chart; limited at shoulder & elbow

A chart or flow sheet should always be dated and signed. For an example of a flow sheet used to supplement notes, see Appendix F.

In certain situations in which the patient has very limited or simple problems, the entire SOAP note may be a flow sheet. See Appendix F for an example of a flow sheet SOAP note format.

Common Mistakes in Recording Objective Data

Some of the most common mistakes in recording objective data are

1. Failure to state the affected part
2. Failure to put things in measurable terms
3. Failure to state the *type* of whatever it is that is being measured or observed

EXAMPLES

(CORRECT)
AROM, the type of ROM measured;
shoulder *flexion*, the type of movement measured;

gait deviations, the type of deviations observed;
sliding board w/c ↔ mat transfers, the type of transfers observed.

If something cannot be stated in measurable terms, the word *appears* instead of *is* should be used.

EXAMPLE

(CORRECT)
Ⓡ UE strength not formally assessed on this date but appears functional for transfers w/c ↔ mat.

The term *appears* should be used cautiously; third-party payers will not provide reimbursement for intervention that "appears" to be needed.

Some Specifics Regarding Recording Objective Data

Using scales with numerical values showing the value of normal—such as 3/5 strength versus fair strength—is suggested to make the job of those reading the notes for third-party payers somewhat easier. Appendix D includes some suggestions regarding recording objective data to maximize the effectiveness of note writing for third-party payers.

The following are some methods for recording objective data. This list is definitely not all inclusive. You can ask your instructors for more specifics about recording objective data as you learn methods of testing and measurement. Also, Appendix E contains references on various methods of measuring and recording objective data.

Edema: Circumferential measurements
Pitting: 0–4+ system of recording
Endurance: Vital signs (BP, respirations, pulse) before treatment, after treatment, and recovery times
Signs of fatigue
Activity (describe) and amount of activity tolerated (time)
Perceived exertion scale
Gait analysis:
Always include: Type of assistance
Equipment needed
WB status
Distance
Include as necessary: Time
Type of surface (level, rough, inclines, stairs, 1-step elevation)
Gait pattern/deviations
General appearance: Atrophy
Skin condition
Thin/obese
Body build
Mental alertness: Oriented x 3 (person, place, time)
Method of transport to PT: Cart/stretcher
W/c
Assistive device
Assistance necessary
Muscle strength: 0–5 system
0–normal system
(Consider using a form or data base sheet)
Substitutions
Alternate positions used for testing (if other than the standard is used)

50

Muscle tone: Increased or decreased tone and where
　　　　　Normal, hypotonic, hypertonic, spasticity, rigidity

Posture: Sitting, standing, supine, prone
　　　　Posterior view, anterior view, side view

Pulse: Beats/minute
　　　Rhythm (regular, irregular)
　　　Beats skipped (if any)
　　　0 through 3+ system of recording

Reflexes: 0 through 3+ or 0 through +++ system of recording
　　　　WNL, ↑, ↓, or absent

Respiration: Pattern
　　　　　Rate
　　　　　Sounds

ROM: (Several methods are taught and used in various facilities)
　　　What restricts (pain, tightness, spasm, edema, loose body, etc.)
　　　Substitutions
　　　Alternative positions (if other than standard used)
　　　Active or passive or active-assisted
　　　cm or degrees
　　　(Consider using a form or data base sheet)

Sensation: Absent, intact, ↑, or ↓
　　　　　Sharp/dull (s/d)
　　　　　Light touch
　　　　　Proprioception/kinesthesis
　　　　　Temperature
　　　　　Deep pressure
　　　　　Stereognosis
　　　　　2-point discrimination

Skin/wounds: Decubiti, rashes, scars
　　　　　Size
　　　　　Color/appearance (pink/red, purplish, slough, eschar)
　　　　　Odor (none, moderate, foul)
　　　　　Undermining
　　　　　Drainage (sero-sanguinous, purulent, green, none)
　　　　　Stages (I–IV)
　　　　　Risk assessment score
　　　　　Pressure relieving device
　　　　　Location

Transfer ability (the following must be included):
　　Type of assistance
　　Type of transfer
　　Equipment needed

Writing Objective Information in Functional Outcomes Reporting

When using functional outcomes reporting with a SOAP note format, often the functional sub-headings are listed first and are emphasized since the purpose is to return patients to an optimal functional status and not to return them to normal strength, ROM, etc. Usually, strength, ROM, sensation, and other nonfunctional headings (physical impairments) follow the functional information and serve as an explanation for the decrease in function. Some facilities use two main categories: *Functional Status* and *Caused By* or *Physical Impairments* and then continue to organize the information in subcategories under these main categories of objective information. The reference list in Appendix E lists several excellent references for functional outcomes reporting in its various formats.

Writing Interim (Progress) Notes

In an interim (progress) note, not every category normally addressed in an initial note will be included. Use only the information obtained while reassessing the patient during treatment sessions.

If a patient's status is unchanged and the area addressed is extremely important, it is acceptable to address the area and state that it is unchanged. However, for the sake of the reader, the unchanged status should be briefly described.

EXAMPLE

(CORRECT)
Transfers: Supine ↔ sit unchanged; still requires mod + 1 assist.

When stating that the patient's status is unchanged, it is important to make sure that all of the evaluation skills and methods available have been used. In the example above, perhaps the amount of assistance needed by the patient is unchanged, but the patient is performing the transfer more quickly (5 minutes to perform the transfer versus 10 minutes).

EXAMPLE

(CORRECT)
Transfers: Supine ↔ sit unchanged; still requires mod + 1 assist. but performance of transfer requires 5 min. on this date (vs. 10 min. initially required). Transfer is becoming more functional.

Data used for comparison purposes can also be included. In the example above, without the comparative data, the fact that the performance of the transfer required 5 minutes would seem insignificant to the reader. The reader may not take the time to look at a previous written note in order to obtain the patient's former status, or the reader may not have the previous note available.

Information addressed in interim notes should include areas addressed in the last set of short term goals written. For example, if a goal is set for the patient to be able to roll supine → sidelying ® independently within 1 week, the patient's rolling status should be addressed under *O* in the next interim note.

As mentioned previously, when writing notes, it is important to know the requirements of both the facility and the third-party payers. In some areas of the country, certain third-party payers require listing both the treatment the patient received and the patient's reaction to the treatment. This can be listed in the *O* part of the note under *reaction to treatment.*

EXAMPLE

(CORRECT)
Reaction to Rx: Pt. received 30 min. of gait training on this date emphasizing correction of gait deviations & correction of balance deficits. Responded well to verbal cues but could not cont. to correct gait deviations s̄ verbal cues

Writing Discharge Notes

The completeness of the *O* section of a discharge note varies greatly among practice settings. In some facilities, the discharge note is similar to an interim note and is an update of the patient's status since the last interim note was written. In other facilities, the discharge note is a more complete summary of the patient's condition upon discharge from the facility and, in format and length, is more similar to the initial note. Still other facilities use a format that summarizes the

52

patient's condition upon beginning therapy, the general course of therapy, and the patient's status upon discharge from therapy.

Types of notes can also vary depending upon who will be reading the note. For example, a note that is forwarded to a nursing home or home health agency might be a complete summary of the patient's condition, whereas a note that will go the medical records storage when the patient is discontinued may simply update the patient's status since the last interim note was written. The home health or nursing home therapist may receive only the discharge summary from an acute or rehabilitation facility, so a more complete note is needed. For the purposes of this workbook, the discharge note is to be considered a complete summary of the patient's status upon discharge and course of therapy, and you are to address all areas of objectives data measured and/or re-measured during treatment.

Summary

The *O* section of the note is a very important section. It should be included in every type of note, whether it is an initial, interim, or discharge note and whether a traditional SOAP format or a SOAP format using functional outcomes as its emphasis is used. The information should be organized under headings, should be written in a clear and concise manner, and should list the results of objective measurement procedures performed by the therapist.

The following worksheets give practice at the skills needed to write the *O* part of a note. Four worksheets are included because this portion of the note includes so many different types of information. After reviewing this chapter, working with the following worksheets, and using the answer sheets to correct the worksheets, you should be able to write the objective portion of a note easily.

Writing Objective (O): WORKSHEET 1

Part I. Mark the statements that should be placed in the *O* category by placing an *O* on the line before the statement. Also mark the *S* items with an *S* and the information that belongs in the Problem portion of the note by writing Prob. on the line before the statement.

1. _____ Will receive pulsed US @ 1.5–2.0 W/cm^2 to Ⓡ upper trapezius.

2. _____ Strength: N throughout all extremities.

3. _____ Pt. has good rehab. potential.

4. _____ Pt. c/o pain Ⓛ ankle.

5. _____ Hip clearing reproduces pain Ⓛ knee.

6. _____ States onset of pain in July 1992.

7. _____ Pt. has been referred to home health services for further Rx.

8. _____ Denies pain c̄ cough.

9. _____ Dx: closed head injury.

10. _____ Transfers: w/c ↔ mat c̄ sliding board c̄ min + 1 assist.

11. _____ Indep in donning/doffing prosthesis within 1 wk.

12. _____ c/o pain Ⓛ low pack p̄ sitting for ~10 min.

13. _____ Will inquire if Pt. can be referred to OT & speech therapy.

14. _____ Gait: Indep c̄ crutches 10% PWB Ⓡ LE for 150 ft. x 2.

15. _____ Pt. was difficult to assess due to lack of cooperation as demonstrated by closing his eyes & crossing his arms when given a command.

16. _____ Will initiate OT post-op per critical pathway.

17. _____ ↑ AROM Ⓡ shoulder to WNL within 2 mo.

18. _____ Rx this date: training in w/c propulsion & management, transfer training c̄ sliding board w/c ↔ mat & sit ↔ supine. Pt. was fatigued p̄ Rx.

19. _____ AROM: WNL bilat LEs.

20. _____ Will be seen by PT as an O.P. beginning c̄ 3x/wk. & progressing prn.

21. _____ States hx of COPD since 1994.

22. _____ Pt. will be indep in dressing & grooming activities within 2 wks.

Part II. Match each *O* statement with the appropriate heading. More than 1 statement may exist for each heading.

    A. Amb
    B. Transfers
    C. Strength
    D. ROM
    E. Sensation
    F. Reaction to Rx

1. _____ UE AROM is WNL except for 0–90° shoulder flexion bilat.

2. _____ ↓ sensation to light touch & pinprick noted in Ⓛ L5 distribution.

3. _____ LE AROM is WNL bilat.

4. _____ Amb is otherwise WNL.

5. _____ Otherwise, UE sensation is WNL.

6. _____ Strength is N in all extremities.

7. _____ Pt. was able to correct his gait $\bar{c}$ verbal cues $\bar{p}$ Rx.

8. _____ Transfers supine ↔ sit are indep but too slow to be functional.

9. _____ Pt. demonstrates ↓ time spent in stance phase on Ⓛ LE & ↓ step length Ⓡ LE.

10. _____ UE sensation is WNL bilat.

11. _____ All other transfers are performed indep & at a normal speed.

Part III. Rewrite the following *O* statements in a more clear, concise, and professional manner. Also, list the heading under which the statement should be placed. (To assist you, an example is given, and some of the problems are in italics in the first few statements.)

EXAMPLE

Passive range of motion is limited to 90 *degrees* of flexion in *both* of her hips.
a. **Heading:** <u>PROM</u>
b. **Corrected statement:** Hip flexion: limited to 90° bilat.

1. The *patient* has *good* strength in *both* of her *arms*.

   a. Heading: _____

   b. Corrected statement: _____

   _____

2. Performing a *straight leg raise* on the *left causes* the *patient's* worst back pain.

   a. Heading: _____

   b. Corrected statement: _____

   _____

3. Strength *is normal* in *right* shoulder *muscles, good* in *right* biceps, *poor* in *right* triceps, *zero* in all other *right* arm musculature distal to the elbow. *Left arm* strength is *normal*.

   a. Heading: _____

   b. Corrected statement: _____

   _____

   _____

   _____

4. Mary *ambulates* for *approximately* 150 *feet full weight bearing with* a walker *twice independently*.

   a. Heading: _____

   b. Corrected statement: _____

   _____

5. The patient was short of breath after transferring supine to sit and bed to bedside chair; her respiratory rate increased from 18 breaths per minute before the transfers to 32 breaths per minute immediately after the transfers.

    a. <u>Heading</u>: _____

    b. <u>Corrected statement</u>: _____

    _____

    _____

    _____

6. Left ankle active range of motion is within the normal range.

    a. <u>Heading</u>: _____

    b. <u>Corrected statement</u>: _____

Part IV. The following are the notes to yourself that you jotted down while performing the objective testing of your patient. (While taking notes for yourself, you did not consult Hospital XYZ's approved abbreviations list.)

UE—strength & AROM—WNL
Gait—independent—walker—NWB Ⓛ LE—50 ft. twice
Ⓛ LE—cast—long leg
Ⓡ LE AROM & strength—normal
Transfers—toilet minimal of 1, sit to and from stand independent, supine to and from sit independent
Curb—(1-step c̄ walker)—minimal of 1
Ambulates in & out of door—min +1—opens & closes door—walker
Ⓛ LE—not assessed further

Rewrite each line into an *O* statement. Include the appropriate category before each statement. (Example: <u>R UE</u>: AROMs WNL except 90° Ⓡ shoulder flexion.)

1. UE—strength & AROM—WNL

    O statement: _____

2. Gait—independent—walker—NWB Ⓛ LE—150 ft. twice

    O statement: _____

3. Ⓛ LE—cast—long leg

    O statement: _____

4. Ⓡ LE AROM & strength—normal

    O statement: _____

5. Transfers—toilet minimal of 1, sit to and from stand independent, supine to and from sit independent

    O statement: _____

6. Curb—(1-step c̄ walker)—minimal of 1

    O statement: _____

7. Ambulates in & out of door—min +1—opens & closes door—walker

    O statement: _____

8. Ⓛ LE—not assessed further

    O statement: _____

Part V. Below you will find headings for the *O* portion of a note. Each is followed by 5 blanks (more than are needed for the exercise). Using the statements from Part IV, write the number of each after its appropriate heading. The statements you list after each heading should be in the order in which they would logically appear in a note (for instance, 1-5-3 may make more sense than if you were to order them 3-1-5).

    A. <u>Amb</u>: _____, _____, _____, _____, _____

    B. <u>Transfers</u>: _____, _____, _____, _____, _____

    C. <u>UEs & Ⓡ LE</u>: _____, _____, _____, _____, _____

    D. <u>Ⓛ LE</u>: _____, _____, _____, _____, _____

Part VI. Using the categories listed above, write the above information into the *O* portion of a note. (Some of the above statements may have to be rewritten to combine similar material into a single statement.) Your partial note should be written to be an acceptable part of the patient's medical record at Hospital XYZ (using approved abbreviations).

O: _____

_____

_____

_____

_____

_____

_____

_____

_____

_____

_____

_____

_____

_____

Answers to "Writing Objective (O): Worksheet 1" are provided in Appendix A.

Writing Objective (O): WORKSHEET 2

Part I. On the first blank line to the left of each statement, mark the statements that should be placed in the *O* category by placing an *O* on the line before the statement. Also mark the *S* items with an *S* and the information that belongs in the Problem portion of the note by writing Prob. on the first line to the left of the statement.

1. _____ DTRs 2+ throughout LEs except 3+ ®̣ KJ.
   _____

2. _____ States was in a car accident & Pt.'s car was hit broadside on the passenger side.
   _____

3. _____ Will request an order for OT to assist c̄ dressing.
   _____

4. _____ Long Term Goal: Independent walker ambulation 150 ft. x 2 FWB within 2 wks.
   _____

5. _____ Amb training, beginning in // bars & progressing to a walker.
   _____

6. _____ Strength testing was difficult because Pt. does not follow commands consistently.
   _____

7. _____ C/o inability to dress indep.
   _____

8. _____ Transfers: Supine ↔ sit c̄ min +1 assist.
   _____

9. _____ X-ray: Osteoporosis.
   _____

10. _____ ↑ PROM Ⓛ knee to 0–90° within 2 wks.
    _____

11. _____ Proprioception: ↓ in entire ®̣ UE.
    _____

12. _____ c/o pain in "entire" Ⓛ UE c̄ or passive movement of the wrist.
    _____

13. _____ AROM ®̣ shoulder flexion ↑ to 0–90° p̄ Rx.
    _____

14. _____ Will be seen BID @ B/S:
    _____

15. _____ Pt. will be given written & verbal instructions in home exercise & walking program.
    _____

16. _____ Sensation: Absent to light touch & pinprick through Ⓛ L5 distribution.
    _____

17. _____ Pt. will demonstrate proper knowledge of back care & ADL by discussion of ADL
_____ c̄ therapist & through 90% correct performance on an obstacle course in back ADL.

18. _____ C/o itching in scar Ⓛ wrist ~2x/hr.
_____

Part II. On the second blank line to the left of each *S* and *O* statement above, mark whether the statement is functional information (mark this by writing Func on the line) or information on physical impairments (mark this by writing Impair on the line).

Part III. Match each *O* statement with the appropriate heading. More than 1 statement may exist for each heading. Place the answer on the first blank line to the left of each statement.

    A. Amb
    B. ADL
    C. UEs
    D. LEs
    E. Trunk
    F. Reaction to Rx

1. _____ LE AROM is WNL bilat except SLR bilat limited to 0–50° due to tight hamstrings.
_____

2. _____ All transfers indep but slow.
_____

3. _____ Tolerated mobilization to lumbar spine, although mobilization to lumbar area is
_____ not pain free.

4. _____ Spasm noted Ⓛ lower lumbar paraspinal musculature.
_____

5. _____ LE strength is WNL bilat except F Ⓛ plantar flexors.
_____

6. _____ Tenderness to palpation in L4-5, L5-S1 area.
_____

7. _____ Pt. tolerated full prone extension exercises well; was able to perform 10 reps s̄ any
_____ reproduction of pain Sx.

8. _____ UE AROMs & strengths WNL.
_____

9. _____ Trunk AROM is WNL; repeated flexion in standing & supine positions ↑ pain in
_____ low back & Ⓛ LE.

10. _____ Posture: ↓ lumbar lordosis, head held in forward position, ↑ thoracic kyphosis.
_____

11. _____ Amb is indep s̄ device but slow c̄ little trunk rotation noted.
_____

12. _____ Ankle jerk 1+ on Ⓛ, 2+ on Ⓡ.

_____

13. _____ SLR + at 45° Ⓛ, − on Ⓡ.

_____

14. _____ Demonstrates improper lifting techniques when asked to lift a box & when asked to transfer pts.

_____

15. _____ LE sensation to light touch & pinprick is diminished in Ⓛ L5 dermatome; otherwise WNL.

_____

16. _____ Repeated trunk extension in standing ↓ pain.

_____

Part IV. On the second blank line to the left of each of the above statements, mark whether the *O* statement discusses Function (write Func on the line) or a physical impairment (write Impair on the line).

Part V. The following are the notes to yourself that you jotted down while performing the objective testing of your patient. (While taking notes for yourself, you did not consult Hospital XYZ's approved abbreviations list.)

1. sit↔stand minimal +1
2. // bars—stood minimal +1 assist—1 min. twice then took 1 step c̄ minimal +1—FWB both LEs
3. LE strength at least F (group muscle assessment)—unable to further assess due to mental status
4. UE strength at least F (group muscle assessment)—unable to assess further due to mental status
5. all ROM WNL except approx 90° shoulder abduction & approx 110° shoulder flexion bilaterally
6. fatigued after standing twice, all other assessment deferred

Place an "X" before the headings you would use to write the *O* portion of this note.

_____ UEs

_____ LEs

_____ trunk

_____ transfers

_____ amb

_____ Rx

_____ endurance

_____ strength

_____ AROM

_____ Ⓡ extremities

_____ ADL

_____ Ⓛ extremities

60

Part VI. Below you will find headings for the *O* portion of the note. (They were chosen because by using them, the information would have to be repeated the least.) Each heading is followed by five blanks (more than are needed for the exercise). Using the notes you wrote above, write the number of each after its appropriate heading. The information you list after each heading should be in the order in which information would logically appear in a note (for instance, 1-5-3 may make more sense than if you were to order them 3-1-5).

    A. <u>Amb</u>: _____, _____, _____, _____, _____

    B. <u>Transfers</u>: _____, _____, _____, _____, _____

    C. <u>Strength</u>: _____, _____, _____, _____, _____

    D. <u>AROM</u>: _____, _____, _____, _____, _____

    E. <u>Endurance</u>: _____, _____, _____, _____, _____

Part VII. Using the categories listed in Part VI above, write the objective information into the *O* portion of a note. Your partial note should be written to be an acceptable part of the patient's medical record at Hospital XYZ (using approved abbreviations).

O: _____

_____

_____

_____

_____

Answers to "Writing Objective (O): Worksheet 2" are provided in Appendix A.

Writing Objective (*O*): WORKSHEET 3

Part I. Below you will find headings for the *O* portion of a note. Each is followed by five blanks (more than are needed for the exercise). Below these headings are seven statements to be included in the note. Write the number of each after its appropriate heading. The statements you list after each heading should be in the order in which they would logically appear in a note (for instance, 1-5-3 may make more sense than if you were to order them 3-1-5). You may wish to write the note out on a separate piece of paper to assist you with this task.

    A. <u>Gait:</u> _____, _____, _____, _____, _____

    B. <u>Transfers:</u> _____, _____, _____, _____, _____

    C. <u>Ⓡ extremities:</u> _____, _____, _____, _____, _____

    D. <u>Ⓛ extremities:</u> _____, _____, _____, _____, _____

1. All transfers are totally dependent.
2. AROM, strength, & sensation WNL throughout Ⓡ UE & LE.
3. Ⓛ UE & LE completely flaccid.
4. No active movement noted in Ⓛ extremities.
5. Sensation intact Ⓛ extremities.
6. Amb not feasible at this time.
7. PROM WNL throughout Ⓛ extremities.

Part II. The following are the notes to yourself that you jotted down during your treatment session while reassessing your patient. (While taking notes for yourself, you did not consult Hospital XYZ's approved abbreviations list.)

propels w/c himself 15 ft. to mat—difficulty getting close to mat & locking brakes—maximum +1
    to place sliding board
maximum +1 to remove armrest
w/c↔mat c̄ sliding board & minimum +1 assist for NWB Ⓡ LE—verbal cues for hand
    placement
sit↔supine c̄ moderate of 1 to move Ⓡ LE
hip flex G Ⓛ, G− Ⓡ
knee flex G Ⓛ
hip abduction bilaterally at least F; not assessed c̄ resistance against gravity
Ⓡ & Ⓛ hip abduction/adduction c̄ 2# x 15 (supine)
Ⓡ & Ⓛ SLR x 15
Ⓛ knee flex c̄ 2# x 15
Ⓛ terminal knee ext c̄ 2# x 15
requires frequent rests

1. Using the categories of your choice, write the above information into the *O* portion of an interim note. Your partial note should be written to be an acceptable part of the patient's medical record at Hospital XYZ.

    O: _____

    _____

    _____

    _____

    _____

    _____

_____

_____

_____

_____

_____

_____

_____

_____

_____

Part III. Using the same information as above, rewrite your note using a functional outcomes reporting SOAP note style.

O: FUNCTIONAL LIMITATIONS: _____

_____

_____

_____

_____

_____

_____

_____

_____

_____

_____

PHYSICAL IMPAIRMENTS: _____

_____

_____

_____

_____

_____

_____

_____

_____

_____

Part IV. Rewrite the following *O* statements in a more clear, concise, and professional manner. Also, list the heading under which the statement should be placed.

1. The patient walks 50 feet twice with 50 percent partial weight bearing on her left leg and requires standby assistance from me to compensate for her vision deficits.

    a. Heading: _____

    b. Corrected statement: _____

    _____

2. Examination of the patient's left ankle reveals two plus pitting edema.

   a. Heading: _____

   b. Corrected statement: _____

3. The knee jerk, when tested, is three plus on the right and two plus on the left.

   a. Heading: _____

   b. Corrected statement: _____

4. John used a sliding board to perform his transfer from the wheelchair to the mat and back requiring my presence to occasionally provide minimal help to stabilize him when he loses his balance.

   a. Heading: _____

   b. Corrected statement: _____

   _____

5. Mary requires two people using maximal assistance to roll her to either side from lying on her back.

   a. Heading: _____

   b. Corrected statement: _____

   _____

Answer to "Writing Objective (O): Worksheet 3" are provided in Appendix A.

Writing Objective (*O*): WORKSHEET 4

Part I. Below you will find familiar headings discussed for the *O* portion of an interim note. Each is followed by five blanks (more than are needed for the exercise). Below these headings are seven statements to be included in the note. Write the number of each after its appropriate heading. The statements you list after each heading should be in the order in which they would logically appear in a note (for instance, 1-5-3 may make more sense than if you were to order them 3-1-5). You may wish to write the note out on a separate piece of paper to assist you with this task.

    A. Gait: _____, _____, _____, _____, _____

    B. Transfers: _____, _____, _____, _____, _____

    C. Strength: _____, _____, _____, _____, _____

1. Sit → stand $\bar{c}$ min +1 assist. & verbal cues for hand placement.
2. Stand → sit $\bar{c}$ mod +1 assist.; pt. does not reach for chair $\bar{a}$ attempting to sit.
3. Amb 100 ft x 3 $\bar{c}$ walker & min +1 assist.
4. Sit → supine $\bar{c}$ standby assist. of 1 & verbal cues.
5. Supine → sit $\bar{c}$ mod assist. of 1.
6. Bilat LE strength grossly 4-/5.
7. Has difficulty turning $\bar{c}$ walker.

Part II. The following is a note written by a student. Using the same information, rewrite this *O* portion of the note using different categories and more concise writing, if and when possible.

O: Appearance: Incision Ⓡ anterior forearm covered $\bar{c}$ steri-strips.
AROM: Ⓡ UE limited shoulder flexion to approx. 120°, abduction to approx. 70°, full elbow flexion, −42° elbow extension, full wrist flexion, wrist extension to neutral $\bar{c}$ full finger flexion. Ⓛ UE full AROM all movements. LEs full AROM all movements.
Strength (gross break test used): Ⓡ UE shoulder flexion fair +, shoulder abduction fair +, elbow flexion & extension good, wrist flexion/extension good, finger flexion & extension good. Ⓛ UE normal all movements. Ⓛ LE good all movements. Ⓡ LE normal all movements.
Sensation: To light touch & pinprick normal all 4 extremities.
Transfers: W/c ↔ mat pivot transfer $\bar{c}$ minimal assist. of 1, sit ↔ supine independent.
Ambulation: $\bar{c}$ walker $\bar{c}$ minimal assist for 50 ft. once wt. bearing as tolerated all extremities.

O: _____

_____

_____

_____

_____

_____

_____

_____

_____

_____

_____

_____

_____

_____

_____

_____

_____

_____

_____

_____

Part III. Using the same information as above, rewrite your note using a functional outcomes reporting SOAP note style.

O: FUNCTIONAL LIMITATIONS: _____

_____

_____

_____

_____

_____

_____

_____

_____

_____

_____

PHYSICAL IMPAIRMENTS: _____

_____

_____

_____

_____

_____

_____

_____

_____

_____

_____

Answers to "Writing Objective (O): Worksheet 4" are provided in Appendix A.

Review Worksheet: Stating the Problem, S, AND O

Part I. Indicate which of the following statements are S statements and which are O statements. Mark them by placing an S or an O on the blank line before the appropriate statement. (Some of the statements are neither S nor O statements.) Also mark the information that belongs in the Problem portion of the note by writing Prob. on the blank line before the statement.

1. _____ Incision healing well, 3 in. in length, located immediately proximal to Ⓛ thumbnail.

2. _____ ↑ AROM Ⓡ shoulder to WNL within 4 wks c̄ 3x/wk. Rx.

3. _____ Will instruct Pt. in a home exercise program to improve posture & alignment (attached).

4. _____ Pt.'s wife states he amb indep s̄ assistive device prior to present hospital adm.

5. _____ DTR's are 2+ throughout.

6. _____ Dx: low back pain.

7. _____ Describes neg. past experience of PT.

8. _____ C/o Ⓡ LE pain in posteriolateral aspects of Ⓡ thigh down to the knee; intensity of pain: 8 (0 = on pain, 10 = worst possible pain).

9. _____ Will attempt to perform manual muscle test on another date when Pt. is more rested.

10. _____ X-ray shows arthritic spurs in lumbar spine.

11. _____ Pulse rate was 75 ā exercise, 95 immediately p̄ exercise, & 75 beats/min. 3 min. p̄ exercise.

12. _____ Amb s̄ assist. device indep & s̄ deviations.

13. _____ Describes onset of pain immediately p̄ lifting a 50 lb. bag of dog food on 1/1/92.

14. _____ BID: Hot pack to low back for 20 min.

15. _____ Pt.'s rehab potential is poor.

Part II. Rewrite the following S and O statements in a more clear, concise, and professional manner. Also, list the part of the note (S or O) and the heading under which the statement should be placed.

1. The patient complains of left lateral knee pain that comes and goes.

   a. Part of the note: _____ b. Heading: _____

   c. Corrected statement: _____

2. The patient doesn't have as much sensation in the left L5 dermatome.

   a. Part of the note: _____ b. Heading: _____

   c. Corrected statement: _____

3. The patient states a doctor "looked in [his] right knee with a scope" on 2/2/94.

   a. Part of the note: _____ b. Heading: _____

   c. Corrected statement: _____

4. The patient says he had "surgery where they opened up my skull" in February 1994.

   a. Part of the note: _____ b. Heading: _____

   c. Corrected statement: _____

5. Right leg passive range of motion is within normal limits throughout.

   a. Part of the note: _____ b. Heading: _____

   c. Corrected statement: _____

Part III. Here are the notes to yourself that you jotted down while reading the chart and assessing your patient. (While taking notes for yourself, you did not consult Hospital XYZ's approved abbreviations list.)

From the Chart

Diagnosis is fractured right femoral neck 1/12/94. A right hip prosthesis was inserted on 1/14/94.

From the Patient

Pain ® hip while standing
No PT or OT before—no walker or cane before this admission—no tub chair or portable commode currently available at home
Fell at home and hit ® hip on side of bathtub
Lives alone—apartment—elevator—curbs only
Apartment bathroom has a bathtub with a shower and shower curtain
Would like to return home p̄ D/C
(For PTs:) Would like to eventually ambulate independently s̄ device once again
(For OTs:) Would like to be able to manage grooming and dressing by herself but would "settle" for Meals on Wheels

From the PT Objective Testing

UEs—ROMs WNL except −5° ® elbow extension
UEs—strength G+ throughout (group muscle test)
ROMs WNL in left leg
® LE—ROMs limited secondary to post-op restrictions to 90° hip flexion, full AROM hip abduction, 0° hip internal and external rotation, 0° adduction
Ⓛ LE—strength G+ throughout (group muscle test)
® LE—strength at least F throughout—not further assessed due to recent surgery
Transfers: w/c ↔ mat moderate + 1
          sit ↔ stand minimal + 1
          supine ↔ sit moderate + 1
Ambulated // bars minimal + 1 approx. 20 feet once 50% PWB ® LE—felt dizzy and nauseated—sent to room—nurses notified

From the OT Objective Testing

UE strength G+ throughtout (group muscle test)
UE—AROM WNL except −5° ® elbow extension
Fine motor skills within functional limits for activities of daily living skills
Tranfers supine ↔ sit with moderate of 1 without use of bedrail
Transfers wheelchair ↔ bed with moderate of 1
Patient initially seen bedside for assessment of grooming skills
Currently has IV infusing in left forearm
Patient able to bathe UEs and trunk but needs minimal assistance of 1 for both LEs and needs set-up for sponge bath
Able to groom her hair independently
Able to care for her teeth independently
Wears contact lenses; able to care for lenses by herself from a wheelchair

Write the above information into the Problem, *S*, and *O* portions of either a physical therapy note or an occupational therapy note. Your partial notes should be written to be an acceptable part of the patient's medical record at Hospital XYZ.

_____

_____

_____

_____

_____

_____

_____

_____

_____

_____

_____

_____

_____

_____

_____

_____

_____

_____

_____

_____

_____

_____

_____

_____

_____

_____

_____

_____

_____

_____

_____

_____

_____

_____

_____

_____

_____

_____

_____

_____

_____

_____

_____

_____

_____

Part IV. Using the same information as above, rewrite your favorite of the two notes using a functional outcomes reporting SOAP note style.

_____

_____

_____

_____

_____

_____

_____

_____

_____

_____

_____

_____

_____

_____

_____

_____

_____

_____

_____

_____

_____

_____

_____

_____

_____

_____

_____

_____

_____

_____

_____

_____

_____

_____

_____

_____

_____

_____

_____

_____

Answers to "Review Worksheet: Stating the Problem, S, and O" are provided in Appendix A.

8 Writing Assessment (*A*): I—The Problem List

The problem list is part of the Assessment (*A*) section of the note. This list provides a summary of the patient's major problems as written in the Subjective and Objective parts of the note. It is not included in the notes at every facility, but some facilities now require it. It becomes a reference point for other healthcare professionals, third-party payers, and others who read the medical record and need a quick overview of the patient's therapy problems, just as we look to the physician's impressions for a summary of the patient's significant medical problems.

Relationship to *S* and *O*

The problem list includes the major areas that were not within normal limits (WNL) when the subjective interview and objective testing were performed. It is usually written in a list format. The steps to formulating the problem list are as follows:

1. (Prerequisite step:) Write the *S* and *O* portions of the note.
2. Review the *S* and *O* portions of the note, jotting down or highlighting findings that are not WNL and that can be influenced or changed by therapy intervention. Medical or psychiatric problems may be part of the physician's problem list and may be listed in the problem area of the note (before *S*), but they do *not* belong in the therapy problem list. Discussion as to how medical or psychiatric problems affect the patient's potential or actual performance in therapy should be included in the *summary* or discussion part of the Assessment section of the note.
3. Set priorities as to which problem is the most important, the next important, and so forth. It is important to remember that the area of setting priorities involves judgment on the part of the therapist. Different therapists may set the priorities differently, depending upon the setting in which they practice, the individual patient's insurance coverage, and so forth. For example, not every therapist would set the priorities for the patient in the example given below in the same order that they have been set.
4. List the physical therapy problems in order of priority.

For example, in this initial note step 1 already completed:

Dx: Degenerative arthritis Ⓡ knee. Ⓡ total knee replacement on (date).

S: <u>C/o:</u> severe pain c̄ AROM Ⓡ knee. <u>Hx:</u> States hx of arthritis Ⓡ knee. <u>Prior level of function:</u> Amb indep s̄ device PTA. Denies previous use of any type of assistive device. <u>Home situation:</u> States lives c̄ his wife. Describes 1 step s̄ handrail to get into Pt.'s 1 story home; states all floors are carpeted except the bathroom. <u>Pt.'s goal/lifestyle:</u> Pt. is a carpenter & would eventually like to return to his job. <u>Pt.'s immediate goal:</u> to function indep at home c̄ crutches.

O: <u>AROM:</u> Ⓡ knee 30–45°. All other joints of UEs & LEs WNL. <u>Strength:</u> Ⓡ LE: 1+/5 quadriceps, 2/5 Ⓡ hamstrings within limited AROM, Ⓡ gastrocnemius not assessed but is able to plantar flex throughout AROM. All other Ⓡ LE musculature of 4+/5 strength. Ⓛ LE & UE: Musculature of 4+/N strength throughout. <u>Transfers:</u> Sit ↔ stand & w/c ↔ mat (pivot) c̄ mod +1 assist. Supine ↔ sit c̄ min +1 assist. for moving Pt.'s Ⓡ LE. <u>Amb:</u> In // bars 10% PWB Ⓡ LE for ~10 ft. x 2 c̄ mod +1 assist. & verbal cues.

(Step 2:) Looking at the *S* and *O* parts of the note, the patient has several problems. They are: pain c̄ AROM Ⓡ knee; ↓ AROM Ⓡ knee; ↓ strength Ⓡ quadriceps & hamstrings; dependence in transfers; dependence in ambulation; and ↓ endurance.

(Step 3:) Although an increase in AROM is a primary need of most patients with total knee replacements, they must first become functional in ambulation and transfers. If absolutely necessary, a patient who is independent in transfers could go home in a wheelchair and become independent in ambulation with further treatment. Therefore, transfers become the greatest priority, with ambulation the second priority. With functional ambulation and transfers, a patient can receive outpatient or home care therapy to increase the knee AROM (the third priority). Typically, an increase in AROM is accompanied by an increase in strength (the fourth priority). Endurance will increase as the patient becomes more independent in all ADL, so endurance is the lowest priority.

(Step 4:)

A: Problem List

1. dependence in transfers
2. dependence in amb
3. ↓ AROM Ⓡ knee
4. ↓ strength Ⓡ quadriceps & hamstrings
5. ↓ endurance during amb

Notice that the problems are listed in functional terms, if possible, and are listed in a general manner, since this list is a summary of the more specific details included under *S* and *O*.

Relationship to Long Term Goals or Expected Functional Outcomes

Usually each problem listed in the note is covered by a long term goal or expected functional outcome. Long term goals are written to describe how each of the problems in the problem list will be finally resolved. Expected functional outcomes list the functional level that the patient is expected to reach by the time he or she is discharged from therapy. Therefore, expected functional outcomes address functional patient problems from the problem list. You will learn more about writing long term goals and functional outcomes in the next section of this workbook.

A Word about Interim Notes and Discharge Summaries

In the interim note, a problem is usually only listed if it is a new problem, if it has been resolved, or if you are referring to the problem. When writing the discharge summary, it is important to note whether a problem has been resolved or still exists.

Summary

While the problem list is not included in the notes of every facility, it is an important part of planning for patient care. It summarizes the information reported in the *S* and *O* sections of the note which is *not* WNL. Judgment is involved in writing the problem list. It helps the therapist to set priorities. It becomes the basis for goal setting.

The worksheets that follow will guide you through the process of formulating a problem list. You will not be expected to recognize abnormal *S* and *O* findings without guidance, nor will you be expected to set the priorities as to which problem is more important without help. After reviewing the above information, completing the worksheets, and comparing your answers to the answer sheet, you should be able to write the problem list portion of the note appropriately, if you are given assistance to recognize the therapy problems and set priorities among them.

Writing Assessment (A): I—The Problem List: WORKSHEET 1

Part I. Here is the note written on a patient.

Dx: Fx Ⓡ femoral neck (date). Ⓡ hip prosthesis inserted (date).

S: C/o: pain Ⓡ hip while standing. Hx: States fell at home & hit Ⓡ hip on side of bathtub. States has had no therapy previously. Home situation: States lives alone in an apartment that is accessible by elevator. Has carpets & needs to amb curbs. Prior level of function: Lived indep PTA & amb s̄ assist device. Pt.'s goals: Short term to return to home c̄ granddaughter staying c̄ her until Ⓡ hip is healed. Long term to return to former lifestyle, amb s̄ assist device.

O: UEs & Ⓛ LE: Transfers: w/c ↔ mat pivot & supine ↔ sit c̄ mod +1 assist. Sit ↔ stand c̄ min +1 assist. Amb: // bars c̄ min +1 assist. ~20 ft x 1 c̄ 50% PWB Ⓡ LE. Pt. became pale & vomited p̄ ~20 ft. of amb; nursing floor was notified & Pt. was returned to her room immediately. AROM: WNL except Ⓡ elbow extension = −5°. Strength: 4+/5 throughout (group muscle test performed). Ⓡ LE: AROMs WNL. Strength at least 3/5 throughout; not further assessed on this date due to recent surgery.

A: Problem list:

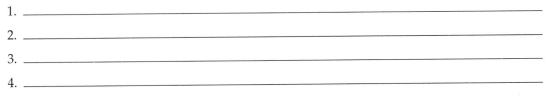

1. _____

2. _____

3. _____

4. _____

Now formulate the problem list:

   A. Look at the *S* part of the note under c/o. You will notice one of the patient's problems. Write the problem here:

   _____.

   B. Look at the section on UEs & Ⓛ LE under *O*. You will notice a problem with elbow extension. Write this problem here:

   _____.

   C. You will also notice that the strength is *not* N. Assume this patient is 83 years old. 4+/5 strength in the unaffected extremities is functional for a person 83 years old. You would therefore not list this as a problem.

   D. Look at the section on Ⓡ LE. As far as you can tell, all is functioning within normal limits. You won't write anything from this section into your problem list because the patient has no real problem in this area.

   E. Transfers: The patient is *not* independent. Write this problem *clearly* and concisely here:

   _____.

   F. Amb: Look at the patient's ambulatory status. Is she independent? If not, write the problem here:

   _____.

Setting Priorities

To achieve the patient's goals, the patient must be able to transfer and ambulate. The patient's transfer ability is the more vital skill area needed for functioning at home. Write these problems into your problem list as problems numbers 1 and 2. The problem with pain will decrease as the patient begins to move around during ambulation and transferring; however, pain can impair movement during transfers and ambulation. The problem of −5° elbow extension existed prior to the patient's recent injury. It is a minor problem and has not interfered with function to this point. Therefore, the elbow extension problem is the least important problem. Write the third and fourth problems into the problem list above.

Part II. The following are the notes to yourself that you jotted down while reading the chart, interviewing and testing your patient. (While taking notes for yourself, you did not consult Hospital XYZ's approved abbreviations list.)

From the Chart

CHF
Hx of ASHD
Hx of degenerative arthritis

From the Subjective Interview

c/o—generalized weakness
      —fatigue
no further assessment—due to mental status

From the Objective Tests Performed

oriented—person—yes
            —place—no
            —time—no
            —date—no
at times combative and argumentative
sit to/from stand c̄ minimal +1 assistance
LE & UE strength at least 3/5 (group muscle test)—unable to further assess—mental status
LE AROM PROM WNL
UE AROM & PROM WNL except ~ 90° shoulder abduction & ~100° shoulder flexion noted
      bilaterally
AROM = PROM
FWB—// bars then stood 1 min x 2—minimal of 1 assistance
fatigue p̄ standing x 2—other assessment deferred—mental status

Write this information into the Problem, *S*, and *O*, parts of a note.

_____

_____

_____

_____

_____

_____

_____

_____

_____

_____

_____

_____ —

_____

_____

_____

Here is the note written thus far. (Note: There are several correct ways in which you could have written this note.)

Dx: CHF; hx of ASHD, degenerative arthritis.

S: c/o: generalized weakness & fatigue. Hx/home situation/prior level of function & goals: Not assessed due to mental status.

O: Transfers: Sit ↔ stand c̄ min +1 assist.
Strength: LE & UE strengths at least 3/5 as per group muscle assessment; unable to further assess due to mental status.
AROM & PROM: All WNL UEs & LEs except ~90° shoulder abduction & ~100° shoulder flexion bilat.
Amb: Stood FWB in // bars 1 min x 2 c̄ min +1 assist.
Endurance: Fatigue p̄ standing x 2; all other assessment deferred.
Orientation: Oriented to person, confused to place, date, time; at times combative & argumentative.

A: Problem list:

1. _____

2. _____

3. _____

4. _____

Now formulate the problem list:

A. Look at the *S* part of the note. Are the patient's complaints something that will be verified in the objective part of the note (*O*)? (Inasmuch as they are, you will wait to look at the objective categories of the note before addressing them in the problem list.)

B. Transfers: Is the patient independent in transfers? If not, write the problem here:

_____.

C. Strength: Is strength specifically a problem? (You can't tell at this point, and you can't further assess this in the usual manner because of the patient's confused mental status. Therefore, you do *not* need to list this as a problem at this time. If it proves to be a problem later for the patient, you can add it to the problem list.)

D. ROM: This is not within normal limits. However, the importance of this problem depends on the patient's lifestyle and her needs for full active shoulder flexion and abduction bilaterally. For now, write it here:

_____.

E. Amb: Look at the patient's ambulatory status. The patient is obviously not independent in ambulation. Write this problem here:

_____.

F. Endurance: This is mentioned under both *S* and *O* as a problem. Write the problem here:

_____.

G. Orientation: The patient's orientation and mental status may prevent the patient from progressing in therapy. While this is a problem, it is not one that therapy can resolve. (Whether or not to include mental status in the problem list is a controversial topic among therapists. It may depend upon whether you are a physical or an occupational therapist and whether you are involved in a reality orientation program.)

78   Setting Priorities

1. The patient must be able to transfer in order to be functional, even in a home situation in which someone cares for the patient. Write this as problem number 1 above.

2. Ambulation is a functional skill that would be very advantageous for the patient to have before returning home. Write this as problem number 2 above.

3. This patient's endurance definitely has to increase, and an increase in endurance goes along with functional ambulation in this case. Write this as problem number 3.

4. The patient's ROM is decreased and may or may not impair function, depending upon her lifestyle. Considering her level of mental functioning, her ROM is probably not a serious problem but should be listed nonetheless. This problem should be listed as number 4, and the level of influence this problem has on function should be further investigated with one of the patient's family members.

Answers to "Writing Assessment (A): I—The Problem List: Worksheet 1" are provided in Appendix A.

Writing Assessment (A): I—The Problem List: WORKSHEET 2

Part I. The following are the notes to yourself that you jotted down while reading the chart, interviewing and testing your patient. (While taking notes for yourself, you did not consult Hospital XYZ's approved abbreviations list.)

From the Chart

Fx proximal ® femur on (date)
ORIF (date) c̄ long plate and screws
17 year old ♀

From the Subjective Interview

c/o dizziness while standing—subsided p̄ 2–3 periods of standing
c/o severe pain (8 on 1–10 pain scale, 10 = worst pain) incision site
c/o difficulty moving ® LE
fell off horse (date)—"landed on my leg wrong"
no assistive device prior to admission
lives c̄ parents & 2 older siblings
4 steps at home to get in, carpeting throughout—bedroom on 1st floor
very active in horseback riding and organizations at school
her goal (short term)—ambulate 17 steps c̄ crutches plus long distances to go back to school as
    soon as possible after discharge
her goal (long term)—return to horseback riding

From the Objective Tests Performed

UE AROM WNL
UE strength N throughout
Ⓛ LE AROM WNL
Ⓛ LE strength N throughout
® LE AROM WNL
® LE strength—N in ankle musculature—at least F in hip and knee musculature (not further
    assessed due to recent surgery)
supine to sit: independent
sit to supine: minimal +1
sit to/from stand in //bars—minimal +1
w/c to/from mat—minimal +1
stood only—// bars—NWB ® LE—~2 min x 3—minimal +1
BP: 1st try—110/70 before standing
            80/40 immediately after standing
            110/70 3 minutes after return to sitting
    2nd try—110/70 before standing
            90/50 immediately after standing
            112/72 3 min after return to sitting
    3rd try—110/72 before standing
            105/68 immediately after standing
            110/70 3 minutes after return to sitting

Write this information into the Problem, *S*, and *O* parts of a note.

_____

_____

_____

_____

_____

_____

_____

_____

_____

_____

_____

_____

_____

_____

_____

_____

_____

_____

_____

_____

_____

_____

For purposes of consistency, the note written thus far is located on the last page of this worksheet. Please refer to it as you continue to work on this worksheet.

A: Problem list:

1. _____

2. _____

3. _____

Now formulate the problem list:

A. Look at subjective findings. Keep these in mind to see if they are addressed in the *O* part of the note. (Two of the areas are addressed in the *O* part of the note. If they are not, you would need to add them to the problem list. Pain is not addressed elsewhere.) Write the problem here:

_____ .

B. UEs & Ⓛ LE: Is anything abnormal? (Since there is not, no comments on these extremities will be included in the problem list.)

C. Ⓡ LE: Is anything abnormal? (We do not know the strength of the right hip and knee musculature, *but* it cannot be assessed any further. All areas assessed were as within normal limits as possible for the patient at this time; therefore, no right lower extremity problems will be included in the problem list.)

D. Transfers: Is anything abnormal? (The patient needs assistance with several transfers.) Write the problem here:

_____.

E. Amb: Is anything abnormal? (The patient is not independent in gait.) Write the problem here:

_____.

F. Vital signs. Is anything abnormal? (Her blood pressure stabilized when she stood the last time, so this is no longer a problem; therefore, this would *not* be included in the problem list.)

Setting Priorities

1 and 2. The patient is not independent in ambulation and transfers. Although both transfers and ambulation are important and functional in nature, transfers would be the priority because they are a more basic functional skill. (Note: Other therapists might disagree.) Write these two problems into your problem list as number 1 and number 2.

3. Pain is a lesser priority than ambulation or transfers. It will decrease with the passing of time and with the patient's participation in functional activities. Write this as problem number 3 in the problem list.

Part II. Using the same information as above, rewrite the above notes using a functional outcomes reporting SOAP note style. (Hint: Remember the only problems listed are functional problems.)

_____

_____

_____

_____

_____

_____

_____

_____

_____

_____

_____

_____

_____

_____

_____

_____

_____

_____

_____

_____

_____

_____

_____

_____

_____

_____

_____

_____

_____

_____

_____

_____

_____

Answers to "Writing Assessment (A): I—The Problem List: Worksheet 2" are provided in Appendix A.

Here is the note written thus far:

Problem: 17 y/o ♀ c̄ a dx of fx Ⓡ proximal femur on (date). ORIF c̄ long plate & screws on (date)

S: C/o: Pt. c/o dizziness on standing which subsided p̄ 2–3 periods of standing. C/o severe pain at incision site (8 on 1–10 scale, 10 = worst pain). C/o difficulty moving Ⓡ LE. Hx: States fell off a horse on (date) & "landed on my leg wrong." Never used any sort of assist. device PTA. Home situation: Lives c̄ parents & 2 older siblings. Describes 4 steps at entrance of 1 story home & carpeting throughout. Prior level of function: States was very active in horseback riding & in various organizations in school. Pt. goals: (Short term) to ambulate 17 steps c̄ crutches plus long distances to be able to return to school ASAP p̄ D/C. (Long term) to return to horseback riding.

O: UEs & Ⓛ LE: AROM WNL. Strength N throughout. Ⓡ LE: AROM WNL. Strength N in ankle musculature & at least F in musculature controlling the hip & knee; hip & knee not further assessed due to recent surgery. Transfers: Supine → sit indep, sit → supine, sit ↔ stand in // bars, & w/c ↔ mat c̄ min +1 assist. Amb: Stood in // bars NWB Ⓡ LE for ~2 min x 3 c̄ min +1 assist. Vital sings: BP readings as follows:

Attempt #	ā Standing	Immediately p̄ Standing	3 Minutes p̄ Return to Sitting
1	110/70	80/40	110/70
2	110/70	90/50	112/72
3	110/72	105/68	110/70

Writing Assessment (*A*): **9** II—Long Term Goals and Expected Functional Outcomes

Long term goals are part of the Assessment (*A*) section of the note. They state the final product to be achieved by therapy. Once the problem list is established, the patient's long term goals are set.

Expected functional outcomes are a specialized type of long term goal. This chapter will first address long term goals and then discuss expected functional outcomes.

Reasons for Writing Goals

Goals are written (1) to help you plan the treatment to meet the specific needs and problems of the patient, (2) to prioritize treatment and measure effectiveness, (3) to assist with monitoring cost effectiveness (for purposes of third-party payment), and (4) to communicate the therapy goals for the patient to other healthcare professionals.

The Structure of a Goal

Before writing long term goals specifically, it is necessary to know the ABCs of writing objectives. Like an educational objective, a good goal for patient care contains four elements:

A. Audience (who will exhibit the skill)
B. Behavior (what the person will do)
C. Condition (under what circumstances—the position, the equipment, and so forth that must be provided or be available for the patient to perform the behavior)

D. Degree (how well will the behavior be done—number of feet, number of repetitions, muscle grades, degrees of ROM; i.e., the amount of improvement you want to see *specifically*).

AUDIENCE

Almost always the patient is the audience. However, it can be a family member or the patient with a family member, as in "Pt. c̄ his wife will be indep in amb stairs & curbs s̄ assist device." Often the audience is implied in goal writing, and it is not necessary to say "Pt. will demonstrate . . . ." or "Pt. will be . . . ."

The audience is *never* the therapist. Goals are patient oriented, not therapist oriented.

BEHAVIOR

This is always a verb, often followed by the object of the behavior. Frequently with long term goals, this is a functional behavior. The object of the behavior must be something that can be *measured* or *described accurately* so that you can document when these goals are achieved. An example is "Pt. will *demonstrate head control* 100% of the time." (Behavior: demonstrate; object of the behavior: head control.)

Sometimes the behavior is implied and not specifically stated. For example, "Indep *amb & transfers* to provide Pt. indep mobility within his home." (Unstated behavior: demonstrate; object of the behavior: ambulation and transfers.)

Behaviors are always stated using *action verbs*. Verbs such as "be" or "know" do not describe observable or measurable activities and, therefore, are not acceptable. Instead, verbs such as demonstrate, list, and state are acceptable.

CONDITION

This includes the circumstances under which the behavior must be done or the conditions necessary for the behavior to occur. An example is "Indep *walker* amb *on level surfaces & curbs* for unlimited distances within 3 wks. to allow Pt. indep mobility at home." A walker, level surfaces, and curbs must be available in order for the patient to perform this type of ambulation.

Sometimes the circumstances under which the behavior must be done are implied. If "Normal pain-free Ⓡ LE AROM & strength" is set as a goal, it is implied that you must have a goniometer available and strength will be measured via manual muscle testing.

DEGREE

This is usually the portion of the goal that is the longest. It includes the minimal number (Example: 40 ft.), the percentage or proportion (Example: 3 out of 4 times), any limitation or departure from a fixed standard (Example: strength to 4/5 within one half grade), or any distinguishing features of successful performance (Example: Ⓡ LE strength equal to Ⓛ LE strength as measured by the Cybex).

When writing goals, the degree of performance must be *realistic, measurable,* or *observable;* must name a specific *time span* in which the goal will be achieved; and must be *expressed in terms of function,* when possible. Discussion of the inclusion of functional terms and the setting of a time span follows in the sections below.

Notice the example of a goal given previously: "Indep walker amb on level surfaces & curbs *for unlimited distances* (measurable) *within 3 wks.* (time span) *to allow Pt. indep mobility at home* (functional terms)."

An analysis of all of the parts of the same goal follows: "Indep walker amb on level surfaces & curbs for unlimited distances within 3 wks. to allow Pt. indep mobility at home."

A. Pt.
B. will amb (demonstrate ambulation)
C. walker (must be present)
   on level surfaces & curbs (these surfaces must be available)

    D. for unlimited distances (measurable)
       Indep (observable)
       within 3 wks. (time span)
       to allow Pt. indep mobility at home (functional)

Another example is "↑ Ⓡ elbow extension AROM to −10° within 2 wks. to improve Pt.'s ability to reach in her overhead cabinets at home."

    A. Pt.
    B. will ↑ Ⓡ elbow extension AROM
    C. it is assumed that a goniometer will be available
    D. −10° (measurable)
       within 2 wks. (time span)
       to improve Pt.'s ability to reach in her overhead cabinets at home (functional)

Functional Terms

Some facilities do not add the final phrase to the goal to put it in functional terms. The advantage of using the final phrase in the example above is to notify third-party payers of the functional reasons for the goal. Using the example above, among professionals it is generally known that the patient will not be very functional in reaching in the overhead cabinets with an elbow with very little AROM; however, this is not always so clear to others.

    It is generally quite important that long term goals state the outcomes of therapy in functional terms since the ultimate goal of therapy is to make the patient more functional.

Time Span

Long term goals are the functional goals for the patient that have a time span of a week, a month, a year, or longer—depending on the patient's diagnosis and general condition and the therapeutic setting. The time span set is the total length of time during which the therapist will see the patient. For example, in an acute care setting, a patient may be seen for only 3 to 5 days, whereas in certain long term pediatric settings, a patient may be seen for a year or longer.

    SETTING THE TIME SPAN. Setting a specific time span for your long term goals is difficult, especially for a new practitioner, since it takes clinical experience to know how quickly a patient will progress. Even experienced therapists cannot always accurately predict the amount of time needed to achieve a goal. Remember, long term goals can be revised if your patient cannot reach the goal within the time span set. Team meetings, clinical instructors, staff members, and class notes can serve as references for setting long term goals while gaining experience. Be patient with yourself as you learn to set realistic time spans.

Clarity

Poorly written goals do not clearly communicate the purpose of your treatment. Some examples of poorly written goals are listed below. Each poorly written goal is compared to one correct version of the goal. (There are many possible correct versions of each poorly written goal below.)

EXAMPLE

POORLY WRITTEN	CORRECTLY WRITTEN
↑ ROM	↑ Ⓡ shoulder flexion AROM to 0–180° p̄ 2 wks. to enable Pt. to return to gymnastics competition.
↓ Pain	↓ Low back pain intensity to 5 on a pain scale (0 = no pain, 10 = worst possible pain) p̄ 10 days of Rx to ↑ pt.'s ability at to sit 4 hrs. at work.

Improve gait pattern	Pt.'s gait pattern $\bar{c}$ prescription AFO will be WNL $\bar{c}$ equal wt. bearing bilat LEs $\bar{p}$ 1 wk. of gait training to decrease Pt.'s rate of falling.
↓ Swelling ® ankle	↓ ® ankle circumferential measurements by 1 cm/measurement at the level immediately inferior to the malleoli to ↑ Pt.'s indep in gait.
↑ General strength	↑ General strength of UEs to 4/5 throughout bilat $\bar{p}$ 2 wks. of Rx to improve Pt.'s ability to lift cooking pots & pans when she cooks.
Promote functional use of ® extremities	↑ Active movement of ® UE & LE out of abnormal synergy patterns to improve use of ® UE & LE during feeding skills & gait.
Indep amb	Indep amb $\bar{c}$ straight cane $\bar{c}$ good knee control for ~100 ft. x 2 to enable Pt. to walk from bedroom to kitchen.
↑ Endurance in amb	Improve functional amb distance to 40 ft. x 2 $\bar{c}$ use of O_2 $\bar{s}$ abnormal ↑ in BP during amb to enable Pt. to walk from kitchen to bathroom & back.
Proper transfers	Pt. will perform indep sliding board transfers w/c ↔ mat $\bar{c}$ correct placement of sliding board, removal & placement of armrest, & use of brakes 100% of the time.
Maintain ROM/strength	Prevent ↓ in UE AROM & strength needed to keep Pt. indep in w/c propulsion & management.

Each of the incorrect goals is missing a time span, a *specific* measurement of the expected outcome of therapy (Example: ↑ ROM to what?), and a functional outcome of the goal. Some are also missing information that clearly defines the goal (Examples: type of ROM, location of the pain).

Revision

Occasionally, long term goals may require revision if (1) the patient's condition changes and will not allow progression to the functional level originally set, (2) the patient's condition changes and allows progression beyond the functional level originally set, or (3) the time span set is no longer appropriate and should be revised.

Relationship to the Problem List

Once the interview and testing of a patient are complete (*S* and *O* portions of the note), the patient's major problems are identified in the problem list. For each of these problems, a long term goal is set. It is acceptable for one long term goal to address more than one problem from the problem list. It is also important to consider the portion of the patient interview regarding the patient's goals when setting long term goals. To use a previous example, the following is an initial note that you wrote:

Dx: Degenerative arthritis Ⓡ knee. Ⓡ total knee replacement on (date).

S: c/o: severe pain c̄ AROM Ⓡ knee

Hx: States hx of arthritis Ⓡ knee. Denies previous use of any type of assist. device.

Home situation: States lives c̄ his wife. Describes 1 step s̄ handrail to get into his 1-story home. States all floors are carpeted except the bathroom.

Pt.'s goals/prior level of function: Pt. is a carpenter & would eventually like to return to his job. Pt.'s immediate goal: to function indep at home c̄ crutches.

O: AROM: Ⓡ knee 30–45°. All other joints of UEs & LEs WNL.

Strength: 1+/5 Ⓡ quadriceps. 2/5 Ⓡ hamstrings within limited AROM. Ⓡ gastrocnemius not assessed but is able to plantar flex throughout AROM. All other Ⓡ LE musculature of 4+/5 strength. Ⓛ LE & UE musculature of 4+ to 5/5 strength throughout.

Transfers: Sit ↔ stand & w/c ↔ mat (pivot) c̄ mod +1 assist. Supine ↔ sit c̄ min +1 assist. to move Pt.'s Ⓡ LE.

Amb: In // bars 10% PWB Ⓡ LE for ~10 ft x 2 c̄ mod +1 assist. & verbal cues.

A: Problem list:

1. Dependence in transfers.
2. Dependence in amb.
3. ↓ AROM Ⓡ knee.
4. ↓ Strength Ⓡ quadriceps & hamstrings.
5. ↓ Endurance during amb.

The long term goals (what will be achieved by the time the patient is discharged from the hospital in 1 wk.) are as follows:

1. Indep transfers on/off toilet, supine ↔ sit, sit ↔ stand, chair ↔ bed so Pt. is safe for ADL at home within 3 wks. (This covers Problem 1.)
2. Indep walker amb FWB Ⓡ LE for at least 150 ft. x 2 on level surfaces & on 1 step elevation so Pt. can function indep in amb at home within 3 wks. (Covers Problems 2 & 5.)
3. ↑ AROM Ⓡ knee to 5–90° within 3 wks. to provide adequate AROM for indep amb. (Covers Problem 3.)
4. ↑ Strength Ⓡ quadriceps & hamstrings to at least F within available AROM within 3 wks. to provide adequate strength for indep amb. (Covers Problem 4.)

Setting Priorities

Long term goals are listed in order of priority in the same way that priorities are set for the problem list. Often, if the priorities for the problem list are set and have at least one long term goal to correspond with each problem on the list, then the long term goals will be in order of priority. For the purposes of this workbook, you will not be expected to set goal priorities. You will be guided on what the goals should be and how to set priorities if the goal priorities are different from the priorities of the problem list.

Relationship to Short Term Goals

Short term goals are written as steps along the way to achieving the long term goals.

EXAMPLE

LONG TERM GOAL

Indep amb c̄ a walker FWB Ⓡ LE for at least 150 ft. x 2 on level surfaces & on 1 step elevation within 1 mo. to allow Pt. to amb around her house.

SHORT TERM GOAL
Pt. will amb 30 ft. x 2 in // bars 10% PWB ⓡ LE within 3 days c̄ min +1 assist.

SHORT TERM GOAL (Later on in the Patient's Progress)
Pt. will amb c̄ a walker 50 ft. x 2 10% PWB ⓡ LE within 1 wk. c̄ min +1 assist.

Short term goals will be thoroughly addressed in Chapter 10. If the patient will not be seen long enough to require both long and short term goals, no short term goals are set. The long term goals are usually referred to simply as *goals* when no short term goals are set for the patient.

Expected Functional Outcomes

As stated previously, expected functional outcomes are a type of long term goal. In a functional outcomes format of SOAP notes, the long term goals are sometimes referred to as expected functional outcomes. Also, all long term goals (or expected functional outcomes) address function. Goals regarding strength or ROM are not the focus and are not stated. It is assumed that the therapist will take care of problems with ROM, strength, and so forth to the extent that is needed to address the patient's functional problems. The focus is on what the patient can and cannot do because of the patient's physical impairments, and *not* on the physical impairments themselves.

A Word About Interim Notes

When writing an interim note, long term goals are usually not addressed unless they have been achieved or need to be revised.

A Word About Discharge Summaries

When writing a discharge summary, list the long term goals and most recent short term goals, indicating which goals have been achieved and which have not been achieved. This is particularly important for long term goals because long term goals by definition list the functional status the patient is to achieve by discharge from therapy.

Summary

Long term goals state the long term plans for the patient. It is important that they are structured and clearly defined. They are based on the therapy problem list and are the basis for setting of short term goals. Long term goals require the clinical judgment of the therapist in order to set the parameters of each goal. Expected functional outcomes are long term goals used in functional outcome reporting that address the patient's functional status only.

The worksheets that follow will assist you in setting long term goals and give you practice in writing the goals. They will also let you analyze several goals, letting you see how each goal is structured correctly. After you review the above material, complete the worksheets, and compare your work to the answers in Appendix A, you should be able to write a long term goal correctly when given the parameters, recognize when a goal is incomplete, and state the components missing from an incomplete long term goal.

Acknowledgment

Instructional Objectives, by the Teaching Improvement Project Systems for Health Care Educators (Center for Learning Resources, College of Allied Health Professions, University of Kentucky, Lexington, KY, 40536-0218) was very helpful in the preparation of this chapter.

Writing Assessment (A): II—Long Term Goals: WORKSHEET 1

Part I. In each of the following examples, identify (A) audience, (B) behavior, (C) condition, and (D) degree. Answer the question after each problem as to whether the long term goal would be included in a functional outcomes reporting format SOAP note.

1. Indep, unlimited w/c use & management at home within 3 mo.

   A. _____

   B. _____

   C. _____

   D. _____

   _____

   _____

   _____

   Would this goal be included in a functional outcomes reporting format?

   _____yes, _____no

2. Within 2 wks. Pt. will demonstrate indep amb c̄ prosthesis s̄ device on at least 14 stairs & for at least 1/2 mi. on even & uneven surfaces to assure Pt.'s ability to amb in & out of his home & around his yard.

   A. _____

   B. _____

   C. _____

   D. _____

   _____

   _____

   _____

   _____

   Would this goal be included in a functional outcomes reporting format?

   _____yes, _____no

3. Pt. will demonstrate full pain-free AROM of the trunk within 4 wks. to prevent further injury while lifting, bending, & turning on his job.

   A. _____

   B. _____

   C. _____

   D. _____

   _____

   _____

   _____

   Would this goal be included in a functional outcomes reporting format?

   _____yes, _____no

4. Pt. will demonstrate segmental rolling $\bar{p}$ 1 yr.

A. _____

B. _____

C. _____

D. _____

_____

Would this goal be included in a functional outcomes reporting format?

_____yes,   _____no

Part II. Given the following components of a goal, write them into a long term goal.

1. A. Pt.
   B. will amb (will demonstrate ambulation)
   C. c̄ a walker, on level surfaces & 1 step elevation, NWB Ⓛ LE
   D. indep (observable)
      p̄ 2 wks. (time span)
      40 ft. x 3 (measurable)
      to allow Pt. to get around her house for ADL (functional).

   Long Term Goal: _____
   _____
   _____
   _____
   _____

2. A. Pt.
   B. will demonstrate care & wrapping of her residual limb
   C. c̄ elastic wrap
   D. indep (observable)
      correctly (observable)
      100% of the time (measurable)
      to prepare for prosthetic training (functional)
      within 2 wks. (time span)

   Long Term Goal: _____
   _____
   _____
   _____
   _____
   _____

3. A. Pt.
   B. will ↑ Ⓡ shoulder flexion and abduction AROM
   C. (assumes you have a goniometer present to measure AROM)
   D. to 120° (measurable)
      within 2 mo. (time span)
      to improve Pt.'s ability to reach items on the shelves in her kitchen & closets at home during ADL (functional)

   Long Term Goal: _____
   _____
   _____
   _____
   _____

4. A. Pt.
   B. will demonstrate pursed lip breathing pattern
   C. during amb and performance of daily exercise program
   D. correct use of breathing pattern (observable)
      100% of the time (measurable)
      to ↑ her efficiency & ability to perform all ADL

   Long Term Goal: _____
   _____
   _____
   _____
   _____

Part III. Write the appropriate long term goals as described below.

A: <u>Problem list:</u>
1. ↓ ability of Pt. to lift the pots & pans in her kitchen
2. ↓ ability of Pt. to reach items in her overhead kitchen cabinets
3. ↓ Ⓡ elbow flexion AROM
4. ↓ Ⓡ biceps strength

Formulate a long term goal for each problem identified and answer the questions after each problem.

1. <u>Problem:</u> ↓ ability of Pt. to lift the pots & pans in her kitchen c̄ her Ⓡ UE. You judge that it will be equal to that of the Ⓛ UE (Pt. is right-handed) within 1 month.

   <u>Long Term Goal:</u> _____
   _____
   _____
   _____

   Would this goal be included in a functional outcomes reporting format?

   _____yes, _____no

2. <u>Problem:</u> ↓ ability of Pt. to reach items in the overhead cabinets of her kitchen. You judge that it will be equal to that of the Ⓛ UE within 1 month.

   <u>Long Term Goal:</u> _____
   _____
   _____
   _____

   Would this goal be included in a functional outcomes reporting format?

   _____yes, _____no

3. <u>Problem:</u> ↓ Ⓡ elbow flexion AROM. You judge that it will increase to −3 to −5 degrees WNL within 2 months.

   <u>Long Term Goal:</u> _____
   _____
   _____
   _____

   Would this goal be included in a functional outcomes reporting format?

   _____yes, _____no

4. <u>Problem:</u> ↓ Ⓡ biceps strength. Presently, Ⓡ biceps strength is F−. You judge that it will be G to N within 2 months.

   <u>Long Term Goal:</u> _____
   _____
   _____

   Would this goal be included in a functional outcomes reporting format?

   _____yes, _____no

Answers to "Writing Assessment (A): II—Long Term Goals: Worksheet 1" are provided in Appendix A.

Writing Assessment (A): II—Long Term Goals: WORKSHEET 2

Part I. In each of the following examples, identify (A) audience, (B) behavior, (C) condition, and (D) degree. Answer the question after each problem as to whether the long term goal would be included in a functional outcomes reporting format SOAP note.

1. Indep amb c̄ straight cane for 150 ft. x 2 on level surfaces & on at least 5 stairs within 2 wks. so Pt.'s level of indep at home ↑'s.

   A. _____

   B. _____

   C. _____

   D. _____

   _____

   _____

   Would this goal be included in a functional outcomes reporting format?

   _____yes, _____no

2. ↑ Ⓛ ankle AROM to WNL within 1 mo. of Rx to return Pt. to prior level of functioning at work.

   A. _____

   B. _____

   C. _____

   D. _____

   _____

   _____

   Would this goal be included in a functional outcomes reporting format?

   _____yes, _____no

3. Pt.'s wife will indep transfer Pt. w/c ↔ supine in bed & w/c ↔ toilet giving min +1 assist. p̄ 2 mo. of Rx & 5 sessions of family teaching.

   A. _____

   B. _____

   C. _____

   D. _____

   _____

   _____

Part II. Given the following components of a goal, write them into a long term goal.

1. A. Pt.
   B. will demonstrate sitting balance
   C. the Pt. is sitting on the edge of a mat undisturbed
   D. good balance (observable)
   for at least 5 min. (measurable)
   p̄ 2 mo. of Rx (time span)
   to allow Pt. to transfer better (goal is a functional goal)

   Long Term Goal: _____

   _____

   _____

   _____

   _____

94

2. A. Pt.
   B. will demonstrate transfers supine ↔ sit, sit ↔ stand, on/off toilet c̄ raised toilet seat
   C. toilet c̄ raised toilet seat & some surface (mat or bed) on which to lie are necessary
   D. independent (observable)
      p̄ 2 wks. of Rx (time span)
      (goal is a functional goal)

Long Term Goal: _____

_____

_____

_____

_____

3. A. Pt.
   B. will explain rationale for & importance of performing AROM exercises daily
   C. (it is assumed that Pt. knows AROM exercises)
   D. p̄ 1 wk. of Rx (time span)
      correctly (observable)
      in order to speed Pt.'s rate of recovery (functional explanation)

Long Term Goal: _____

_____

_____

_____

4. A. Pt.
   B. will demonstrate w/c propulsion
   C. on level surfaces including tiled and carpeted surfaces
   D. independently (observable)
      after two months of treatment (time span)
      to ↑ Pt.'s independence at home (functional)

Long Term Goal: _____

_____

_____

_____

_____

Part III. Write the appropriate long term goals as described below.

Case

You have just completed the *S* and *O* portions of a note.

A: Problem list:
1. abnormal gait pattern.
2. ↓ Ⓛ hip AROM.
3. ↓ strength of Ⓛ hip musculature.

Long Term Goals:

1. _____

_____

2. _____

_____

3. _____

_____

Formulate a long term goal for each problem identified.

1. Problem: abnormal gait pattern.
   You judge that this will be normal within 2 months. This is important because the patient is young and walked s̄ deviations ā her injury. Write the long term goal in the space provided above.

2. Problem: ↓ (L) hip AROM.
   You judge that this will increase to within normal limits within 1 month. This will enable the patient to return to her gymnastics class. Write the long term goal in the space provided above.

3. Problem: ↓ strength of (L) hip musculature.
   You judge that this will increase to 4–5/5 within 2 months. This will also enable the patient to return to her gymnastics class. Write the long term goal in the space provided above.

Part IV. Now rewrite the problem list and long term goals into a functional outcomes reporting SOAP note format. (Hint: The problems will be worded the same; however, only functional problems are listed. The same is true for the expected functional outcomes—formerly long term goals.) Remember to include her return to sport in the expected functional outcomes.

A: Problem list:

_____

_____

_____

Expected Functional Outcomes:

_____

_____

_____

Answers to "Writing Assessment (A): II—Long Term Goals: Worksheet 2" are provided in Appendix A.

10 Writing Assessment (*A*): III—Short Term Goals

Short term goals are part of the Assessment (*A*) portion of the note. They are the interim steps along the way to achieving long term goals (which are the final product of therapeutic intervention). Once the expected final outcomes of therapy (long term goals) have been determined, the short term goals are then set. The specific treatment regimen is designed to achieve the short term goals.

In a functional outcomes reporting SOAP format, the short term goals address only function. This chapter will address short term goals and then discuss the differences found in a functional outcomes reporting format.

Reasons for Writing Goals

Goals are written (1) to direct treatment to the specific needs and problems of the patient, (2) to prioritize treatment and measure the effectiveness of treatment, (3) to assist with cost effectiveness (for purposes of third-party payment), and (4) to communicate therapy goals to other healthcare professionals. Short term goals help to guide the immediate treatment plan. Periodically reviewing and resetting short term goals helps the therapist and the patient realize the progress that the patient has made.

The Structure of Short Term Goals

Like long term goals, short term goals are objectives and need to contain the elements that a good objective contains:

A. Audience
B. Behavior

C. Condition
D. Degree

A brief review of the definitions of the elements of a goal with examples from short term goals follows.

AUDIENCE

Almost always, the audience is the patient. However, it *can* be a family member, as in "Pt.'s wife will indep wrap pt.'s residual limb c̄ 3-in. elastic wrap c̄ verbal cues only within 1 wk." Often the audience is implied in goal writing, and it is not necessary to say "Pt. will demonstrate . . ." or "Pt. will be . . . ."

BEHAVIOR

This is always indicated by a verb followed by the object of the behavior. Good examples are " ↑ AROM . . . ," " ↓ dependence in dressing . . . ," and "improve gait pattern . . . ." The object of the behavior must be something that can be *measured* or *described accurately* so that an increase can be documented at a later date.

CONDITION

This includes the circumstances under which the behavior must be done. Examples are " ↓ dependence in *walker* amb to min +1 assist. within 1 wk.," "indep amb s̄ *assistive device on level surfaces* for 10 ft. x 2 within 1 wk."

As with long term goals, the circumstances under which the behavior must be accomplished are sometimes implied. An example of this would be manual muscle testing. Unless otherwise stated, if a muscle grade is set as a goal, it is assumed that the standard testing positions and protocol are used.

DEGREE

This includes the minimal number, the percentage or proportion, any limitation or departure from a fixed standard, or any distinguishing features of successful performance.

When writing goals, the degree of performance must be *realistic, measurable,* or *observable,* name a specific *time span,* and be *expressed in terms of function,* when possible.

Consider the example of a goal given previously: "Pt.'s wife will wrap Pt.'s residual limb c̄ 3-in. elastic wrap c̄ *verbal cues only* (measurable) *within 1 wk.* (time span) *to prepare the pt. for prosthetic training* (functional terms)."

Review this goal and analyze its parts: "Pt.'s wife will wrap Pt.'s residual limb c̄ 3-in. elastic wrap c̄ verbal cues only within 1 wk. to prepare Pt. for prosthetic training."

A. Pt.'s wife
B. Wrap Pt.'s residual limb
C. 3-in. elastic wrap is necessary
D. c̄ verbal cues only (observable)
    within 1 wk. (time span)
    to prepare Pt. for prosthetic training (functional)

Another example follows: " ↑ AROM Ⓡ knee flexion to 5–55° within 3 days to improve Pt.'s transfers & gait."

A. Pt. (implied)
B. will ↑ Ⓡ knee flexion AROM
C. no conditions given (assumed: goniometer will be used)

D. 5–55° (observable)
within 3 days (time span)
to improve Pt.'s transfers & gait (functional)

Functional Terms

Therapists at some facilities do not add the final phrase to the goal to put it in functional terms. The advantage of using the final phrase in the examples above is to notify third-party payers of the functional reasons for the goal. Among professionals it *is* generally known that the patient will not be very functional in transfers and ambulation with a knee with very little AROM; however, this is not always so clear to others. The goal of wrapping the residual limb is not always clear to all medical personnel working with the patient and certainly could confuse third-party payers if this is one of the patient's major goals. Including functional terms is becoming increasingly more normative when writing all goals.

If an explanation of a goal is needed and stating the goal in functional terms is not adequate enough to explain the reasons for setting the goal, it should be explained further under the *Summary* or *Impressions* section under Assessment (*A*).

Although short term goals are not written using functional terms as often as are long term goals, the importance of using functional terms is rapidly increasing. Some therapists assume that if the long term goals are functional and the short term goals correspond well with the long term goals, then the functional reasons for the short term goals are obvious. However, the relationship between the long term goals and short term goals is not as obvious as therapists may assume. Other therapists always use function and only state functional short term goals (in a functional outcomes reporting SOAP note format). This varies from facility to facility. You will adapt your style of writing goals as you adapt to various clinical settings.

Clarity

Poorly written goals do not clearly communicate the purpose of treatment. If certain components of a well-written goal are not included (such as the time span, functional terms, or measurable terms), the purpose of treatment may be very unclear. The lack of clarity will be especially confusing to third-party payers and healthcare professionals who are not familiar with therapy treatment techniques and their purposes. At times, the goal must be related to patient function for the purpose of therapy to be clear to those reading the patient care note.

Time Span

Short term goals are patient objectives that have a time span for their achievement. This can be a few days or a week or longer, depending on the patient's diagnosis and general condition. For example, a patient with a traumatic brain injury may take 3 to 4 months for rehabilitation at times, so short term goals can be set weekly or occasionally for a 2-week period of time. Other patients in long term care settings or pediatric patients may have long term goals set for 1 year and short term goals may be set for 1 to 3 months.

SETTING THE TIME SPAN. Setting a specific time span in which a goal will be achieved is difficult, especially for new practitioners, since it takes clinical experience to know how quickly a patient will progress. At times even experienced clinicians have difficulty predicting how quickly a patient should progress. Generally, a clinician can consider when a note on a particular patient must be written again and what the patient's status will be at that time. If the patient's status will change by the time a note is due to be written, the time span can be set to correspond with the date the note is due. If achieving the goal will take longer, choose a longer time span. If it will take less time, set a shorter time span. Remember: Short term goals can always be revised if the time span set is not correct. Clinical instructors, peers, and class notes can serve as references for setting realistic time spans.

Short term goals are not necessary at times because of an anticipated extremely short patient length of stay. For example, if the patient is only to be seen by therapy one or two times, the long term goals or expected functional outcomes are adequate and short term goals are not needed.

Usually, if the patient is to stay less than 2 weeks, short term goals are not set. Often, if short term goals are not set, the long term goals may be referred to as "goals" instead of "long term goals."

Revision

Short term goals must be revised periodically. A short term goal should be revised if (1) the time period mentioned in the goal has passed, or (2) the patient has achieved the goal set. Consider a previous example:

↓ dependence in walker amb to min +1 assist. for 10 ft. x 2 within 1 wk. to facilitate indep walker amb at home.

Assume 3 days have passed and the patient requires minimal +1 assistance and is progressing. The goal is reset to read:

↓ dependence in walker amb to standby assist. for 60 ft. x 4 within 1 wk. to facilitate amb functional distances needed for home.

Another week passes and the patient's rate of progress has decreased. The therapist now comments on lack of progress and resets the goal:

"Goal to ↓ amb dependence not yet achieved due to . . . (It is good to give a reason if there is one.) Will ↓ dependence in amb c̄ a walker to standby assist. for 60 ft. x 4 within 1 more wk. of Rx.

Relationship to Long Term Goals

Short term goals are based on the patient's long term goals.

EXAMPLE

LONG TERM GOAL (PEDIATRIC PATIENT)
Pt. will propel her w/c for ~100 ft. on tiled & low-pile carpeted surfaces c̄ verbal cues only p̄ 1 yr. of Rx to facilitate indep mobility of pt. at school.

SHORT TERM GOALS
1. Pt. will move UEs out of abnormal synergy patterns in gravity-eliminated planes within 2 mo. of Rx to enable pt. to propel her w/c.
2. Pt. will propel her w/c for ~10 ft. on tiled surfaces only c̄ occasional min +1 assist. & verbal cues within 2 mo. of Rx to facilitate indep mobility at school.

SHORT TERM GOALS (LATER ON IN PATIENT'S PROGRESS)
1. Short term goal #1 of (date) achieved. New short term goal #1: Pt. will move UEs out of abnormal synergy patterns in gravity-resisted planes within 2 more mo. of Rx to enable pt. to propel her w/c.
2. Short term goal #2 of (date) achieved. New short term goal #2: Pt. will propel her w/c for ~10 ft. on tiled surfaces c̄ verbal cues only within 2 mo. of Rx to facilitate indep mobility at school.

Setting Priorities

In the same way that priorities are set for the problem list and long term goals, short term goals should be listed in order of priority. If the short term goals correspond well to the long term goals and the long term goals are listed in order of priority, frequently the priorities for the short term goals will not have to be reset. For the purposes of this workbook, you will not be expected to set

100

goal priorities. You will be guided in setting the goals and in setting goal priorities if the priorities of the short term goals are different from those of the long term goals or if there are two or more short term goals that correspond to one long term goal.

Relationship to the Treatment Plan

When short term goals are set, the therapist (with the patient's input) determines the course treatment will take for the next few days. When a treatment plan is set up, some sort of treatment to work toward *each* of the short term goals must be included.

EXAMPLE

A: <u>Long term goals:</u>

1. Indep walker amb on level surfaces FWB for 70 ft. x 2 & on 1-step elevation within 3 wks. so pt. can get in & out of her home & amb within her home.

2. ® quadriceps strength of at least F within 3 wks. to ↑ indep in amb.

<u>Short term goals:</u>

1. Amb c̄ walker 50% PWB ® LE for ~20 ft. x 2 within 1 wk. to facilitate amb at home (from 1st long term goal above).

2. Pt. will indep demonstrate exercises that he is to perform in the hospital room within 2 Rx sessions to ↑ amb indep (from 2nd long term goal above).

3. Pt. will demonstrate ® quadriceps strength of at least P within 1 wk. to ↑ amb indep (from 2nd long term goal above).

P: <u>BID in PT dept</u>: Amb training c̄ a walker, beginning c̄ 50% PWB & progressing wt. bearing & distance as tolerated (from 1st short term goal). Pt. will be given written & verbal instruction in exercise program to be performed in the hospital room (attached) (from 2nd short term goal). AAROM progressing to AROM exercises ® knee, emphasizing quadriceps functioning (from 3rd short term goal).

Further explanation of the relationship of the treatment plan to the short term goals is discussed in Chapter 12.

Short Term Goals and Functional Outcomes SOAP Format

Facilities differ in their use of short term goals with a functional outcomes SOAP format. Some facilities do not use short term goals because they believe the expected functional outcomes guide treatment sufficiently without short term goals. Other facilities use short term goals that are functional in nature and correspond exactly to the expected functional outcomes. Still other facilities use short term goals that address the physical impairments (decreases in range of motion, strength, and so forth) needed to attain the expected functional outcomes.

Short Term Goals in Interim (Progress) Notes

When writing an interim note, the therapist refers to the short term goals and sets new short term goals if the previously set short term goals have been achieved. If a short term goal previously set has not yet been achieved, the therapist comments on the reason it has not yet been achieved and either resets the goal to make it more reasonable or restates the goal as a goal to be achieved by the next interim note to be written.

1. "Short term goals: Goal #4 of (date) not yet achieved due to ↓ in patient's medical status; will cont. to work toward same goal for 1 more wk."
2. "Short term goals: All achieved. Will work directly toward long term goals set on (date)."

Short Term Goals in Discharge Notes

When writing a discharge summary, the therapist may comment on the most recently set short term goals as to whether or not they were achieved and why. However, in a discharge summary the emphasis should be on the long term goals and why they were or were not achieved. At some facilities, no comment is made on the short term goals in the discharge note because it is assumed that during the patient's final few days or week(s) of therapy, the patient should be working toward the long term goals.

Summary

Setting short term goals is the third step in the assessment and planning process for the patient. Short term goals are based on the long term goals and direct the immediate course of the treatment plan. The time period covered by short term goals is briefer than that for long term goals. Revision of short term goals is done on a regular basis and generally indicates that the patient is making progress. Setting short term goals involves professional judgment.

The worksheets that follow will assist you in setting short term goals and give you practice in writing the goals. They will also let you analyze several goals, allowing you to see how each goal is structured. After reviewing the above material, completing the worksheets, and comparing your work to the answers in Appendix A, you should be able to write a short term goal correctly when given the parameters of the goal, recognize when a goal is incomplete, and state the components missing from an incomplete short term goal.

Acknowledgment

Instructional Objectives, by Teaching Improvement Project Systems for Health Care Educators (CENTER FOR LEARNING RESOURCES, College of Allied Health Professions, University of Kentucky, Lexington, KY 40536-0218), was very helpful in the preparation of this chapter.

Writing Assessment (A): III—Short Term Goals: WORKSHEET 1

Part I. In each of the following examples, identify the audience (A), behavior (B), condition (C), and degree (D). Answer the question after each problem as to whether the short term goal would be included in a functional outcomes SOAP note format.

1. <u>Short term goal</u>: ↑ ⓡ shoulder flexion AROM to 0–90° within 6 Rx sessions to enable Pt. to reach her overhead kitchen cabinet cupboards.

   A. _____

   B. _____

   C. _____

   D. _____

   _____

   Would this goal be included in a functional outcomes reporting format?

   _____ yes, _____ no

2. <u>Short term goal</u>: Pt. will grasp object in midline 3 out of 4 times within 3 mo. in order to increase the Pt.'s functional use of his UEs during ADLs.

   A. _____

   B. _____

   C. _____

   D. _____

   _____

   Would this goal be included in a functional outcomes reporting format?

   _____ yes, _____ no

3. <u>Short term goal</u>: Pt. will demonstrate good body mechanics by correct performance of at least 90% of tasks in obstacle course p̄ 3 Rx sessions in order to prevent further Pt. injury.

   A. _____

   B. _____

   C. _____

   D. _____

   _____

   Would this goal be included in a functional outcomes reporting format?

   _____ yes, _____ no

Part II. Given the following components of a goal, write these into a short term goal.

1. A. Pt.
   B. will ↓ dependence in ambulation
   C. using a walker, on level surfaces only
   D. NWB ⓛ LE, ~100 ft., 1 wk. of Rx independent

   <u>Short Term Goal</u>: _____

   _____

   _____

   _____

   _____

2. A. Pt.'s wife & son
   B. transfer pt. w/c ↔ supine in bed
   C. bed & w/c are necessary
   D. independently
      p̄ 4 family training sessions

Short Term Goal: _____

_____

_____

_____

_____

3. A. Pt.
   B. wrap residual limb
   C. Ace wrap
   D. independently
      5 Rx sessions
      to prepare for prosthetic training

Short Term Goal: _____

_____

_____

_____

_____

Part III. In each of the cases listed below, write the appropriate short term goal and answer the question after each problem.

1. **Case 1**
   O: Donning/doffing prosthesis: Requires verbal cues & mod +1 assist.
   A: Problem list: Dependence in donning/doffing prosthesis.
   Long term goal: Indep donning/doffing prosthesis in 1 wk.

   Short term goal: _____

   _____

   You judge that 1 week from now only standby assistance of one person and no verbal cues will be needed.

   Would this goal be included in a functional outcomes reporting format?

   _____ yes, _____ no

2. **Case 2**
   Dx: Ⓡ CVA.
   O: Amb: Stands in // bars c̄ mod +1 assist. & verbal cues for wt. shift. Wt. shift onto Ⓛ LE is poor; Pt. bears only 10 lbs. of wt. on Ⓛ LE.
   A: Problem list:
   1. Dependence in amb.
   2. ↓ wt. shift onto Ⓛ LE.
      Long term goal:
      1. Indep amb c̄ straight cane for unlimited distances c̄ normal gait pattern, including normal wt. shift onto Ⓛ LE.

   Short term goal: _____

   _____

   You judge that in 1 week minimal assistance of one person and verbal cues will be needed for the patient to be able to stand in the parallel bars with at least half of his body weight shifted onto his left leg.

   Would this goal be included in a functional outcomes reporting format?

   _____ yes, _____ no

3. **Case 3**
   Dx: L4 herniated disc. Lumbar laminectomy performed on (date).
   O: Trunk: Can tolerate lying prone for 5 min. Cannot tolerate further trunk extension.
   Long term goal: Full trunk extension AROM in 1 wk.

Short term goal: _____

_____

You judge that in 2 days the patient will be tolerating the prone-on-elbows position for 5 min.

Would this goal be included in a functional outcomes reporting format?

_____yes, _____no

Part IV. State which components each of the following short term goals are missing.

1. <u>Short term goal</u>: Pt. will be able to perform sliding board transfers.

   Answer: _____

   _____

2. <u>Short term goal</u>: Pt. will demonstrate the correct position for hip flexor stretching.

   Answer: _____

   _____

3. <u>Short term goal</u>: 10-min. exercise routine $\bar{s}$ fatigue within 5 wks.

   Answer: _____

   _____

Answers to "Writing Assessment (A): III—Short Term Goals: Worksheet 1" are provided in Appendix A.

Writing Assessment (A): III—Short Term Goals: WORKSHEET 2 **107**

Part I. In each of the following examples, identify the audience (A), behavior (B), condition (C), and degree (D). Answer the question after each problem as to whether the short term goal would be included in a functional outcomes reporting SOAP note format.

1. Short term goal: $\bar{p}$ 6 Rx sessions, will ↑ cardiopulmonary endurance as demonstrated by max ↑ resp rate of 5 resp/min. $\bar{p}$ amb for 150 ft.

   A. _____

   B. _____

   C. _____

   D. _____

   _____

   Would this goal be included in a functional outcomes reporting format?

   _____yes, _____no

2. Short term goal: Pt. will be able to long sit propped $\bar{c}$ a pillow or wedge maintaining good head position 0–45° of neck flexion for 1 min. within 6 wks. of Rx.

   A. _____

   B. _____

   C. _____

   D. _____

   _____

   Would this goal be included in a functional outcomes reporting format?

   _____yes, _____no

3 Short term goal: Pt. will transfer supine ↔ sit on a mat using rotation & pushing $\bar{c}$ his UEs (1 out of 3 attempts correct) within 2 mo.

   A. _____

   B. _____

   C. _____

   D. _____

   _____

   Would this goal be included in a functional outcomes reporting format?

   _____yes, _____no

Part II. Given the following components of a goal, write them into a short term goal.

1. A. Pt.
   B. hold head
   C. while Pt. is supine
   D. erect in midline, for 15 sec., within 3 mo. of Rx

   Short Term Goal: _____

   _____

   _____

   _____

2. A. Pt.
   B. rolling supine ↔ prone
   C. on a mat
   D. in 6–8 wks., independently

Short Term Goal: _____

_____

_____

3. A. Pt. c̄ minimal assistance from his wife
   B. ambulate stairs c̄ walker
   C. walker & stairs must be available
   D. 5 stairs, 50% PWB Ⓡ LE, independently, 1 wk.

Short Term Goal: _____

_____

_____

_____

_____

Part III. In each of the cases listed below, write the appropriate short term goal.

1. **Case 1**
   Dx: COPD; respiratory failure.
   O: Functional use of UEs: Unable to take any items out of overhead cupboards.
   Strength: F throughout UEs bilat.
   AROM: Limited to 90° bilat.
   Endurance: c̄ 5 reps of both UE PNF diagonals, Pt.'s pulse ↑ by 20 beats/min.
   A: Problem list: ↓ ability of pt. to retrieve items from overhead cupboards
                          ↓ endurance
                          ↓ ROM UEs
                          ↓ UE strength bilat.

   Long term goals:
   1. Pt. will be able to retrieve items less than 1 lb. in weight from lower shelf of overhead cabinet.
   2. Pt. will tolerate 20 reps of both UE PNF diagonals c̄ a rise in pulse of 20 beats/min. or less within 1 mo. of Rx to enable Pt. to use UEs in ADL.

   Short term goals: _____

   _____

   _____

   _____

   You judge that the patient will tolerate 7 repetitions of each of the 2 PNF patterns for the arms after 1 week of treatment.

   Now rewrite the problem list, and the long and short term goals above into a functional outcomes reporting SOAP note format. (Hint: The problems will be worded the same; however, only functional problems are listed. The same is true for the expected functional outcomes [formerly long term goals].)

   A: Problem list:

   _____

   _____

   _____

   Expected functional outcomes:

   _____

   _____

Short term goal:

_____

_____

2. **Case 2**
   Dx: Whiplash.
   S: c/o: neck pain of an intensity of 9 (0 = no pain, 10 = worst possible pain) c̄ any movement of the neck.
   O: AROM: 0–5° cervical rotation Ⓛ & Ⓡ.
   A: Long term goal: ↑ neck AROM to WNL & pain free within 1 mo.

   Short term goal: _____

   _____

   You judge that the patient will be able to move her head to about 10° of rotation to either side in 2 days.

3. **Case 3**
   Dx: Fx Ⓡ tibial plateau. Long leg cast applied (date).
   O: Amb: c̄ walker 40 ft. x 1 NWB Ⓡ LE c̄ mod +1 assist.
   A: Long term goal: Indep amb c̄ crutches for unlimited distances on level surfaces & stairs within 2 weeks of Rx.

   Short term goal: _____

   _____

   You judge that the patient will be able to ambulate 40 ft. twice on level surfaces in 1 wk. but will still require minimal assistance of 1 person to ambulate.

Part IV. State which components each of the following short term goals are missing.

1. Short term goal: ↓ dependence in amb to min +1 c̄ walker 40 ft. x 2 NWB Ⓡ LE.

   Answer: _____

   _____

2. Short term goal: ↑ Ⓡ shoulder abduction AROM within 3 days.

   Answer: _____

   _____

3. Short term goal: ↑ & ↓ stairs c̄ min +1 assist.

   Answer: _____

   _____

Answers to "Writing Assessment (A): III—Short Term Goals: Worksheet 2" are provided in Appendix A.

11 Writing Assessment (A): IV—Summary

What Makes Up the A Part?

The Assessment (A) part of the note contains the analysis of plans and goals for the patient. It involves the professional judgment of the therapist in identifying the patient's problems and setting goals and priorities. Several different kinds of information are included in the assessment part of the note. Each category of information is briefly described below.

PROBLEM LIST

The problem list has already been discussed. See Chapter 8 for more information.

GOALS

Enough has been said already on short and long term goals. See Chapters 9 and 10 for more information.

DRAWING CORRELATIONS/JUSTIFYING DECISIONS

The assessment part of the SOAP note provides an opportunity for the therapist to draw correlations between the S, O, A, and P portions of the note that would not necessarily be obvious to all parties who read patient care notes. Inconsistencies between the patient's complaints and the objective findings can be discussed. Justification for the goals and/or treatment plan can be listed. Comments can be made regarding a patient's progress in therapy and/or his or her rehabilitation potential. Reasoning for information not obtained can be listed. Further testing or treatment needed and/or community services that would be helpful to the patient can be discussed. For the physical therapist, a physical therapy diagnosis, if used in the therapist's work setting, can be listed in this section of the note.

Inconsistencies

In the A portion of the note, the therapist has the opportunity to pinpoint inconsistencies between the S and O findings. (Example: "Although Pt. states she cannot amb well enough to go home, Pt.'s amb status in PT indicates that the Pt. is indep c̄ good endurance.")

Justification for the Goals Set, the Treatment Plan, and/or Clarification of the Problem

The *A* part of a note might include a statement justifying unusual goals. For example, a therapist might get a patient with a diagnosis of CVA who has the potential to transfer independently. However, the patient's wife has been helping to transfer him for years. Both he and his wife are satisfied with the situation and do not want to change the way they have been living. You might then set your goal: "Pt. will perform all transfers c̄ min assist. from his wife within 1 mo." You would comment: "Due to Pt.'s previous functional level of requiring assist. for transfers from his wife, & Pt. & wife's desire to return to the previous functional level only, a goal of indep transfers is not realistic."

The *A* portion of a note could also include justification for further therapy for a patient who initially appears relatively independent. (Example: "Although amb is indep, Pt.'s progress toward indep transfers is slower. Pt. cont. to need assist. c̄ all transfers & lives alone.")

Discussion of Patient's Progress in Therapy

A discussion of the patient's progress in therapy could include further explanation of the patient's failure to progress as quickly as the goals predicted. It could also explain why a patient suddenly regresses or progresses more quickly than anticipated. (Example: Pt. has become more dependent in transfers during the past 2 wks. 2° inactivity associated c̄ pneumonia.)

Patient's Rehabilitation Potential

The *A* part of the note is the opportunity to state whether the patient has rehab potential and why. Some facilities require that every initial note contain a comment about rehab potential. In other settings, an occasional comment may be made regarding rehab potential, but nothing is mentioned regularly.

Difficulty Obtaining Information

The therapist can document whether there was any difficulty obtaining information from the patient and why part of the initial interview and testing could not be performed because of (1) *patient's psychological status* (Example: "Could not accurately assess tone on this date as Pt. cried throughout Rx session."), (2) *lack of willingness to cooperate* (Example: "Could not correctly position Pt. for parts of manual muscle test due to Pt.'s refusal to move out of the supine position."), or (3) *medical problems* (Example: "Unable to measure Ⓛ hip PROM 2° recent surgery.").

Suggestion of Further Testing/Treatment Needed

A therapist can state that a patient might benefit from another service offered within the hospital or in the community (especially if the therapist practices within a setting in which it is not possible to refer the patient directly). The therapist can also state that the patient might benefit in the future from a treatment that is not presently being used (Examples: "Pt. could benefit from OT for training in kitchen ADLs ā returning home alone." "Pt. is a good candidate for the Back School Program once his pain ↓ .").

Testing procedures that would be helpful but could not be completed during the initial therapy session can be listed. (Example: "Further testing of sensation & proprioception is needed.").

Physical Therapy Diagnosis

In some facilities, the therapist states the physical therapy diagnosis. This differs from the medical diagnosis in that the physical therapy diagnosis is a classification *used* to *guide physical therapy treatment* that best fits the patient's signs, symptoms, and functional deficits. Other therapists do not use the term physical therapy diagnosis but may state that the patient's signs/symptoms/functional deficits are consistent with a certain category or classification of patient problem.

There may be some other unusual but significant factor about the patient that should be mentioned. This, too, can be placed under *A*. Make sure that it is not a part of *S* (c/o, Hx, home situation, prior level of function, Pt. goals) or *O* before it is placed in the *A* portion of the note.

How to Actually Write *A*

There is no one set method of writing the information in *A*. It should be *organized* and *easy to follow*. Language should be *professional* and as *clear and concise* as possible.
An example follows:

EXAMPLE

> **A:** Pt. has shown some difficulty in learning home exercise program despite written handout. Therefore, reviews of home program will be needed until Pt. can reach independence.
> Problem list: . . .
> Long term goals: . . .
> Short term goals: . . .
>
> **OR**
>
> **A:** Problem list: . . .
> Long term goals: . . .
> Short term goals: . . .
> Imp (or Summary): Pt. has shown some difficulty in learning home exercise program despite written handout. Therefore, reviews of home program will be needed until Pt. can reach independence.

Summary

The entire *A* portion of the SOAP note is extremely important. It summarizes the *problems* that have been found and *goals* that the therapist thinks the patient can attain to overcome the problems; immediate goals for a short period of time; and a discussion of the findings, correlating and justifying what is written in the *S*, *O*, *A*, and *P* parts of the note. The *A* part of the note, as a whole, requires much professional judgment. Experience will enable the new practitioner to write this section of the note more easily and without assistance.

The worksheets that follow will give you practice writing all of the *A* part of the note. They will help tie the information gained in the previous worksheets on the problem list, long term goals, and short term goals together with the information on correlation described above. After reviewing all of the sections of the workbook involved in the *A* section of the note, completing all of the worksheets, and comparing your work to the answer sheets, you should be able to write the entire *A* portion of the note with assistance in identifying the problems, setting the goals and priorities, and drawing correlations.

Writing Assessment (A): IV—Summary: WORKSHEET 1   **113**

Part I. Mark the statements that should be placed in the *A* category by placing an *A* on the blank line before the statement. Also, mark the *S* and *O* items with an *S* and *O*, and indicate the information that belongs in the problem portion of the note by writing Prob. on the blank line before the statement.

1. _____ <u>Strength</u>: Grossly P (2/5) throughout all extremities.
2. _____ Pt. c/o pain Ⓡ knee.
3. _____ States onset of pain in Dec. 1994.
4. _____ Denies pain c̄ cough or sneeze.
5. _____ Indep in donning/doffing prosthesis within 1 wk.
6. _____ Will enquire if Pt. can be referred to a dietician.
7. _____ Pt. was difficult to test due to lack of cooperation as demonstrated by closing his eyes & crossing his arms when given a command.
8. _____ ↑ AROM Ⓡ shoulder to WNL within 6 wks. to enable patient to reach items in her overhead cabinets.
9. _____ Will be seen 3x/wk. as an O.P.
10. _____ Pt. will demonstrate normal gait pattern within 3 wks. to enable her to amb for functional distances s̄ pain.
11. _____ States hx of COPD since 1990.
12. _____ ↓ sensation noted in C8 distribution.
13. _____ <u>PROM</u>: WNL bilat LEs.
14. _____ Will cont. to attempt to teach home exercise program.
15. _____ <u>Gait</u>: Requires min +1 assist. c̄ crutches 10% PWB Ⓡ LE for 150 ft. x 2.
16. _____ C/o pain Ⓛ low back p̄ sitting for 10 min.
17. _____ <u>Hx</u>: TIA in 1990, ASHD, CHF.
18. _____ Pt. has been referred to home health services for further Rx.
19. _____ Hip clearing reproduces pain Ⓛ knee.
20. _____ Pt. has good rehab potential.
21. _____ Pulsed US underwater at 1.5–2.0 W/cm^2 to Ⓡ wrist.
22. _____ <u>Pt. goals</u>: To return home s̄ assist. p̄ 2 wks. of Rx.

Part II. Of the following *A* statements, identify which statements are part of the problem list (Prob. List), which are short term goals (Short), which are long term goals (Long), and which belong in the rest of the *A* (Summary) part of the note. Note: Each problem from the problem list has a corresponding long term goal and short term goal listed also.

1. _____ Pt. had difficulty following commands because Pt. is hard of hearing.
2. _____ Dependence in transfers.
3. _____ ↑ AROM Ⓡ elbow to 10–55° within 1 wk. to allow Pt. better use of Ⓡ UE in ADLs.
4. _____ Pt. will transfer w/c ↔ mat c̄ sliding board c̄ mod +1 assist. in 1 wk.

114

5. _____ ↓ AROM ® elbow.

6. _____ Pt. has poor rehab potential.

7. _____ Dependence in w/c propulsion & management.

8. _____ ↑ strength ® triceps to G p̄ 1 mo. of Rx to allow Pt. to use her UEs normally during ADLs.

9. _____ N upper abdominal strength within 3 mo. to allow normal movement and posture.

10. _____ States he has had Rx previously; "it has never helped in the past & it will not help now."

11. _____ ↑ AROM ® elbow to 10–110° within 3 wks. to allow patient to functionally feed herself.

12. _____ ↓ upper abdominal strength.

13. _____ Indep w/c propulsion & management within 4 mo. to allow Pt. indep function in her w/c at home.

14. _____ ↑ strength ® triceps to G p̄ 2 wks. of Rx to work toward WNL UE function.

15. _____ F upper abdominal strength in 3 wks. to work toward normal, pain-free posture.

16. _____ ↓ strength ® triceps.

17. _____ Pt. does not respond to therapist verbally or c̄ facial expressions & no family member was present; therefore, subjective interview was not completed.

Part III. Rewrite the following *A* statements in a more clear, concise, and professional manner.

1. The patient has very little chance of wheelchair independence.

   Answer: _____

2. The patient didn't answer or do anything I said because he can't hear well.

   Answer: _____

   _____

3. The patient did not answer any questions straight but always gave an elusive answer while I was trying to do the initial interview.

   Answer: _____

   _____

Answers to "Writing Assessment (A): IV—Summary Worksheet 1" are provided in Appendix A.

Writing Assessment (A): IV—Summary: WORKSHEET 2   115

Part I. Mark the statements that should be placed in the A category by placing an A on the blank line before the statement. Also, mark the S and O items with an S and O and mark the information that belongs in the problem portion of the note by writing Prob. on the blank line before the statement.

1. _____ States was in a car accident & Pt. was thrown from his car.

2. _____ Indep walker amb 150 ft. x 2 FWB within 2 wks. to allow Pt. to amb from her car into her house.

3. _____ Orientation: Pt. is not oriented to date, place, or task & does not follow instructions consistently.

4. _____ Transfers: Supine ↔ sit c̄ min +1 assist.

5. _____ Proprioception: ↓ noted throughout entire Ⓡ UE.

6. _____ Will see BID at B/S.

7. _____ Sensation: Absent to light touch & pinprick throughout C5 distribution.

8. _____ C/o ↓ sensation in fingertips of Ⓛ fingers 2–5.

9. _____ Within 1 wk., Pt. will demonstrate proper knowledge of back care during ADLs by discussion of ADLs c̄ therapist & through passing a practical exam in back ADL.

10. _____ ↓ strength Ⓡ ankle musculature.

11. _____ Pt. will be given written & verbal instructions in home exercise & walking program.

12. _____ C/o pain in "entire" Ⓛ LE c̄ active or passive movement of Ⓛ knee.

13. _____ ↑ AROM Ⓛ knee to 0–90° within 2 wks. to work toward indep rising from chairs & indep stair amb.

14. _____ C/o inability to dress indep.

15. _____ Amb training, beginning in // bars & progressing to a walker.

16. _____ Will request an order for Speech Pathology to assess Pt.'s language abilities.

17. _____ DTRs 2+ throughout LEs except 3+ Ⓡ KJ noted.

Part II. Of the following A statements, identify which statements are part of the problem list (Prob. List), which are short term goals (Short), which are long term goals (Long), and which belong in the rest of the A (Summary) part of the note. Note: Each problem from the problem list has a corresponding long term goal and short term goal listed also.

1. _____ Indep amb s̄ device on level surfaces for 40 ft. x 2 & 4 stairs p̄ 2 wks. of Rx to enable Pt. to amb at home.

2. _____ Pt. is unable to follow commands to hold against resistance during manual muscle test 2° mild confusion.

3. _____ Pt. will transfer supine ↔ sit c̄ min +1 assist. p̄ 1 week of Rx to work toward indep in ADLs.

4. _____ ↓ circumferential measurements of Ⓡ LE by 1 cm at all levels p̄ 4 days of Rx.

116

5. _____ Dependence in transfers.

6. _____ ↓ dependence in amb to min +1 for 10 ft. x 2 in. // bars p̄ 3 days of Rx.

7. _____ Pt. will set up TENS unit c̄ use of written instructions p̄ 1 training session to enable Pt. to perform ADLs s̄ pain.

8. _____ ↑ circumferential measurements Ⓡ LE 2° edema.

9. _____ ↓ circumferential measurements of Ⓡ LE to equal those of Ⓛ LE p̄ 10 days of Rx to ↑ normal use of Ⓡ LE.

10. _____ Pt.'s wife refuses to come to therapy to learn to assist Pt. c̄ transfers so goals for transfer indep c̄ wife will not be achieved.

11. _____ Dependence in use of TENS unit.

12. _____ Indep transfers supine ↔ sit, sit ↔ stand, on/off toilet p̄ 2 wks. of Rx.

13. _____ Pt.'s nausea during the past wk. has inhibited her progress in therapy.

14. _____ Pt. will indep set up & adjust TENS unit for pain control p̄ 3 training sessions to assure indep pain-free ADLs.

15. _____ Pt. could benefit from OT to teach her to dress indep.

16. _____ Dependence in amb.

Part III. Rewrite the following A statements in a more clear, concise, and professional manner.

1. The patient talked so much because of his distractibility that it was difficult to complete the interview.

   Answer: _____

   _____

2. The patient had a bowel movement while ambulating, and therefore there wasn't enough time to finish the initial testing.

   Answer: _____

   _____

3. The patient will be independent in wheelchair propulsion and management but will probably not ambulate.

   Answer: _____

   _____

   _____

Answers to "Writing Assessment (A): IV—Summary: Worksheet 2" are provided in Appendix A.

Review Worksheet: SOA

Part I. Begin by turning to the corresponding answer sheet at the end of these instructions so that you can write your partial SOAP note directly on the answer sheet.

The following are the notes to yourself that you jotted down while reading the chart, interviewing, and performing the objective testing of your patient. (While taking notes for yourself, you did not consult Hospital XYZ's approved abbreviations list nor were you particularly careful in your notation style.)

Write the information into the Problem, *S*, and *O* portions of the note, and the beginning of the *A* portion of the note on the answer sheet. (Further instructions will be provided to help you write the rest of the *A* portion of the note.) Your partial note should be written to be an acceptable part of the patient's medical record at Hospital XYZ.

FROM THE CHART

Diagnosis is: degenerative joint disease Ⓡ hip—total hip replacement on (date)

FROM THE SUBJECTIVE INTERVIEW

Ⓡ hip pain—area of sutures—intensity of 7 when moving—intensity of 3 when sitting (0 = no pain, 10 = worst possible pain)
prior to adm.—intensity of pain was 9 or 10 constantly
1 step at home—railing on Ⓡ going up
owns a 3-in-1 commode, a walker, and a cane
previous left total hip replacement 1/10/94
immediately prior to admission—no assistive device
lives c̄ wife—in his own home
retired—hobby is gardening
plans to return home with his wife after D/C
eventually wants to return to gardening and yard work activities
has not been told about the precautions for patients with total hip replacements

FROM THE OBJECTIVE TESTS PERFORMED

sit to/from stand with moderate of 1
supine to/from sit with minimal of 1
w/c to/from mat pivot with moderate of 1
toilet transfers not assessed
UE AROM WNL
UE strength G+ throughout bilaterally (group muscle test)
Ⓛ LE strength G throughout (group muscle test)
Ⓛ LE AROM WNL throughout
Ⓡ LE—strength grossly T in hip and knee musculature—ankle dorsiflexion G+/N—ankle plantar flexion at least P but not tested further because of the non-wt.-bearing status
Ⓡ LE—AROM—WNL ankle—PROM 0–20° hip flexion, 0–10° hip abduction, 0° hip extension—adduction of hip, internal and external rotation not tested because of hip precautions and recent surgery—knee: 0–70°
incision—10 cm long—staples intact—over greater trochanter Ⓡ—healing well
stood parallel bars moderate of 1—1 min. x 2—10% PWB Ⓡ leg
good rehab potential (your professional opinion)

WRITING A

In writing the assessment portion of the note, follow these directions.
Formulate a problem list based on the *S* and *O* parts of the note.

1. Look at the *S* portion of the note under *c/o*. Write a problem for this.

   Problem: _____

2. Look at the patient's knowledge of precautions for patients with total hip replacements. Write a problem for this.

   Problem: _____

3. Look at the transfer portion of the note. Write a problem for this.

   Problem: _____

4. Look at the section on UE strength (wherever this information is located in the note). While the strength is not N, if the patient is in his 70s, G+ strength can be considered as WNL. Do not write a problem for this.

5. Look at the section on Ⓛ LE strength (wherever this information is located in the note). Write a problem for this.

   Problem: _____

6. Look at the section on Ⓡ LE. Write two problems regarding the Ⓡ LE.

   Problem a: _____

   Problem b: _____

7. Look at the patient's ambulatory status. Write a problem for this.

   Problem: _____

SETTING PRIORITIES

1. Look at function first. Without knowledge of the total hip replacement precautions, the patient could seriously harm his hip and increase his pain during functional activities. Write this as the first problem on the answer sheet.

2. Ambulation and transfers are the most functional problems. Write them as problem numbers 2 and 3 on the answer sheet. (Transfers are needed before the patient can ambulate.)

3. Of the problems with strength, the Ⓛ LE problem may need to be resolved for the patient to be able to ambulate for functional distances and become independent in transfers. Write this problem as number 4 on the answer sheet.

4. As the Ⓡ LE strength increases, the patient's PROM and AROM will increase. Also, the patient's pain will decrease as the Ⓡ LE strength and AROM increase. Because of its influence on so many other problems, write the problem with the Ⓡ LE strength as problem number 5 on the answer sheet. Write the ROM problem as number 6 on the answer sheet.

5. The patient's pain will gradually decrease as the patient heals and the other problems are resolved. This is not to discount the importance of the pain to the patient. The pain levels will decrease relatively quickly as the patient participates in therapy. Therefore, no specific pain management technique is usually used for patients with total hip replacements at Hospital XYZ. List this problem as number 7 on the problem list.

Long Term Goals

Set a long term goal for each problem using the information in the note.

1. The patient does not know the precautions for patients with total hip replacements. You judge that the patient will be able to independently state and demonstrate them within 2 weeks. Write the goal as number 1 on the answer sheet.

2. The patient requires asssistance during transfers. You judge that the patient will achieve independence in 2 weeks (specific transfers listed in your note). Write the goal as number 2 on the answer sheet.

3. The patient requires assistance for ambulation and really cannot ambulate. You judge that the patient will achieve independence in 2 weeks (be sure to check the home situation to include the necessary type of elevation at the entrance to his home). You judge that the patient will be able to use a walker. Write the goal as number 3 on the answer sheet.

4. Ⓛ LE strength is G throughout. You judge that the patient will be able to achieve N (5/5) strength within 2 weeks. Write the goal as number 4 on the answer sheet.

5. The AROM and strength of the right lower extremity are obviously decreased. You judge that the patient will be able to achieve at least fair strength (write it as 3/5 for the sake of the third-party payers) in his hip flexors, extensors, abductors, and adductors within 2 weeks. Write the goal as number 5 on the answer sheet.

6. You judge that the patient will achieve pain-free (see also problem 7 previously) AROM with 0–90° right hip flexion and WNL right hip abduction and right hip extension within 2 weeks. Write the goal as number 6 on the answer sheet.

7. The patient complains of pain in his right hip. The goal set for this was combined with the goal for AROM above.

Short Term Goals

Now set the short term goals based on the list of long term goals.

1. Look at the first long term goal (precautions). Look at what you said about precautions in your note. You judge that the patient will be able to correctly state the precautions whenever asked within 3 days. Write this as the first short term goal on the answer sheet.

2. Look at the second long term goal (transfers). Look at the patient's functional status right now (see your note). First, you judge that the patient will decrease his dependence in sit ↔ stand and w/c ↔ mat to minimal assistance of one person in 3 days. Write this short term goal as number 2 on the answer sheet. You then judge that the patient will be able to achieve transfers supine ↔ sit independently in 1 week. Write this short term goal as number 3 on the answer sheet. You cannot yet set a goal for toilet transfers since you have not yet assessed them.

3. Look at the third long term goal (ambulation). Look at the patient's present status in your note. You judge that the assistance needed for ambulation in the parallel bars will be minimal assistance of one person within 3 days. You also judge that the patient will ambulate 10 feet twice within the same time period. Write this as goal number 4 on the answer sheet.

4. Look at the fourth long term goal (Ⓛ LE strength). Look at the patient's present status. You judge the patient will be able to become independent in an Ⓛ LE exercise program for his room in 3 days. Write a short term goal for this on the answer sheet.

5. Next, you judge it will take 2 weeks for the patient to get N (5/5) strength, but he should be able to demonstrate G+ (4+) in 1 week. Write a short term goal on the answer sheet for this.

6. Look at the fifth long term goal (Ⓡ LE strength). You judge that the patient's strength will be at least P (2/5) in all his right hip and knee musculature within 1 week. Write this goal on the answer sheet.

7. Look at the sixth long term goal (Ⓡ LE AROM). You judge that the patient's AROM will be 0–90° in hip flexion and WNL hip abduction and extension within 1 week. You also judge that the patient will describe his right hip pain as having an intensity rating of 5 with AROM exercises within 1 week. Combine this information and write a short term goal on the answer sheet.

Review Worksheet SOA Answer Sheet

Part II. Use this answer sheet to write the Problem, *S*, *O*, and *A* portions of a note according to the instructions given in the preceding pages. Use additional sheets of paper to complete your note as needed.

Problem List:

1. _____

2. _____

3. _____

4. _____

5. _____

6. _____

7. _____

Long Term Goals:

1. _____

_____

2. _____

_____

3. _____

_____

4. _____

5. _____

_____

6. _____

Short Term Goals:

1. _____

_____

_____

2. _____

_____

3. _____

4. _____

_____

5. _____

_____

_____

6. _____

7. _____

_____

8. _____

_____

_____

Part III. Use this answer sheet to write the Problem, *S*, *O*, and *A* portion of a functional outcomes note using the same information as in the note above. Use additional sheets of paper to complete your note as needed. Hint: The number of blanks left for the Problem List, Long Term Goals, and Short Term Goals may be more than should be needed for a functional outcomes note.

_____

_____

_____

_____

_____

_____

_____

_____

_____

_____

_____

_____

_____

_____

_____

_____

_____

_____

_____

_____

_____

_____

_____

_____

_____

_____

_____

_____

_____

_____

_____

_____

_____

_____

Problem List:

1. _____
2. _____
3. _____
4. _____
5. _____
6. _____
7. _____

Expected Functional Outcomes:

1. _____
   _____
2. _____
   _____
3. _____
   _____
4. _____
5. _____
   _____
6. _____
   _____

Short Term Goals:

1. _____
   _____
   _____
2. _____
   _____
3. _____
4. _____
   _____
5. _____
   _____
6. _____
7. _____
   _____
8. _____
   _____

Answers to "Review Worksheet: SOA" are provided in Appendix A.

Writing Plan (*P*) **12**

The plan portion of the note contains the plan for the patient's treatment. One or more treatments exist to achieve each of the short term goals. Certain information must be included in the plan section of the note, just as certain information is needed in order for the *S* or *O* portions of the note to be complete. Some variations are needed to write the plan section of a discharge note.

Information Included under Plan

The following information *must be* included in the plan section of a note:

1. Frequency per day or per week that the patient will be seen.
2. The treatment the patient will receive. (The amount of specificity may depend on the setting. See below for more detail on describing treatment. For the purposes of these worksheets, a significant level of detail is expected.)
3. If a discharge note, where the patient is going and the number of times the patient was seen in therapy.

The following are also frequently included in the plan section:

4. The location of the treatment (at bedside, in the department, in a pool, at home).
5. The treatment progression.
6. Plans for further assessment or reassessment.
7. Plans for discharge.
8. Patient and family education (e.g., home program plans or what was taught to the patient or the patient's family—attach a copy of any home programs [signed and dated, of course] to the note, if possible).
9. Equipment needs and equipment ordered/sold to the patient (if a discharge note).
10. Referral to other services; if there are plans to consult with the patient's physician regarding further treatment or referral.

An example follows:

EXAMPLE

P: Will be seen 3 x/wk. as an outpatient. Will receive pulsed US to Ⓡ anterior shoulder at 1.5 W/cm² for 5 min. followed by PROM & AROM exercises to Ⓡ shoulder. Exercises will be followed c̄ an ice pack to Ⓡ shoulder for 15 min. Pt. will be instructed in home exercise program for Ⓡ shoulder AROM (attached).

The plan (*P*) portion of the note describes the plan for the patient's treatment (*what the patient will receive*). This differs from the situation of describing the treatment and reaction to treatment in the objective portion of the note. If treatment is addressed in the objective portion of the note, it may include specifics of *what was done with the patient that day and/or the patient's reaction to treatment.*

EXAMPLE

O: <u>Reaction to Rx</u>: Tolerated 10 reps each of quad sets & SLR to (L) LE; c̄ 10th repetition of SLR Pt.'s quadriceps were fatigued & pt. could no longer perform SLR.

P: Cont. c̄ quad sets & SLR 3 x/wk. as an O.P. Will progress to 20 reps as tolerated.

Relationship to Short Term Goals

Once the short term goals are set, a treatment plan is then set up to achieve each of the short term goals. One exercise may achieve more than one goal. In fact, it is advantageous and economically sound to establish the treatment program to achieve the goals most efficiently. When setting up a treatment program, each short term goal, the patient's allotted time for therapy, the patient's endurance level, and the patient's level of boredom must be considered.

EXAMPLE

A: <u>Long term goals</u>:

1. Indep walker amb on level surfaces FWB for 70 ft. x 2 & 1-step elevation within 10 days.
2. (R) quadriceps strength of at least F within 10 days.
   <u>Short term goals</u>:
1. Amb c̄ walker 50% PWB (R) LE for ~20 ft. x 2 within 1 wk. (from 1st long term goal above).
2. Pt. will indep demonstrate exercises that he is to perform in his room within 2 Rx sessions (from 2nd long term goal above).
3. Pt. will demonstrate (R) quadriceps strength of at least P within 1 wk. (from 2nd long term goal above).

P: BID in dept: amb training c̄ a walker beginning c̄ 50% PWB & progressing wt. bearing & distance as tolerated per physician's orders (from 1st short term goal); Pt. will be given written & verbal instruction in exercise program to be performed in his room (attached) (from 2nd short term goal); AAROM progressing to AROM exercises (R) knee emphasizing quadriceps functioning (from 3rd short term goal).

Recording Treatment

Here are some things to consider and include when recording the treatment plan.

Modalities:
  Which modality
  Where
  How long
  Intensity (hot packs: toweling thickness)
  What position (one that is best, most comfortable)
  Examples:
    US: W/cm^2, time, where, position, reaction, coupling agent
    Electrical stimulation: type of current, intensity, type of contraction, where, time, position

Ambulation:
  Distance
  Level of assistance
  Device(s)
  Time
  Wt.-bearing status
  Type of gait pattern
Exercise:
  Extremity or trunk
  Types
  Repetitions
  Position
  Equipment used
  Modifications
  Amount of resistance given (or wt. used)
  Home programs (sometimes attached to D/C notes as part of medical record):
    Brief goal/rationale statement
    Illustrations
    Position
    Directions: keep language simple and in patient terms
    Repetitions and times/day
    Progression
    Equipment
    Precautions

Writing Plan in a Functional Outcomes SOAP Note Format

When writing the plan portion of the note, the therapist documents what he or she plans to do. The treatment plan does not change, no matter which note format is used. Therefore, the plan portion of the note is not different in a functional outcomes SOAP note format.

A Word about Interim Notes and Revision

From time to time, the treatment plan will need to be revised as the patient's condition is reassessed and new short term goals are set. When revision is necessary, the revision of the treatment plan is mentioned in an interim note, along with the changes noted in subjective and/or objective findings and in the goals.

  In some settings, the plan is addressed in every interim note, whether or not there are changes. In the case of no change, a phrase such as "Cont. c̄ previously described program" or "Cont. c̄ same program" is sometimes used.

A Word about Discharge Notes

Generally, the following should be briefly stated:

  1. What the treatment was.
  2. If instruction in a home program was done.
  3. If any other type of instruction was performed.
  4. If the patient was sold any type of equipment (weights, assistive device, lumbar roll, etc.).
  5. If a referral to a home health agency or any other professional was made.

  If instruction of any kind is performed, the following information should be considered or recorded:

  Who was instructed (patient, patient's family member).
  The *type* of instruction (verbal, written, demonstration).

128

The level of the patient/patient's family functioning (could independently demonstrate, could correctly describe the activity, could state the precautions needed for ADL, etc.).

The discharge note should also include:

6. The number of times the patient was seen in therapy.
7. If and when the patient was not seen/on hold and why.
8. Any instances of the patient skipping or canceling treatment sessions.
9. To where the patient is discharged (rehabilitation center, skilled nursing facility, home).
10. The reason for discharge (goals achieved, transfer to another facility, patient requested discharge from therapy, patient's death).
11. Recommendations for follow-up treatment or care given to the patient.

EXAMPLE

P: Pt. was seen BID for gait & transfer training & Ⓛ LE AROM exercises 02-12-94 through 02-15-94. Pt. refused Rx in p.m. of 02-13-94 & a.m. of 02-14-94 2° severe nausea. D/C PT on this date p̄ 6 Rx sessions 2° D/C of Pt. from Hospital XYZ to home. Pt. & Pt.'s daughter were instructed in attached home program & given a copy of same program & Pt. was indep in same program. A walker was ordered for Pt. per Pt. request. Pt. will be followed by ABC Home Health PT.

Summary

The plan (*P*) part of the note is the final step in the planning process for patient care. In initial and interim notes, it outlines the treatment to be used with the patient. In discharge notes, it summarizes the treatment the patient received, the total number of treatments received, any patient education performed, handouts or equipment given or sold to the patient, and recommendations for future treatment or follow up care.

The worksheets that follow give you the chance to identify plan (*P*) statements and to write the plan portion of the note. For the purposes of this workbook, you will not be expected to generate an appropriate treatment plan without guidance. After reviewing the above information, completing the worksheets, and comparing your work to the answer sheets, you should be able to write the plan part of the note if you are given the treatment information to be included.

Writing Plan (P): WORKSHEET 1

Part I. Mark the statements that should be placed in the P category by placing a P on the blank line before each P statement. Also mark the Problem, S, O, and A statements by writing Prob, S, O, or A on the blank line before the appropriate statement.

1. _____ Pt.'s cardiac status may influence his rate of recovery.

2. _____ Pt. has been referred to home health services for further PT & OT Rx.

3. _____ C/o pain Ⓛ ankle c̄ PWB on Ⓛ LE.

4. _____ <u>Strength</u>: T (1/5) in Ⓡ lower trapezius.

5. _____ States onset of pain p̄ a fall in Jan, (year).

6. _____ Indep in donning/doffing back brace within 1 wk.

7. _____ Pulsed US at 1.5–2.0 W/cm² to Ⓡ upper trapezius for 5 min.

8. _____ Pt. c/o constant pain Ⓡ knee of an intensity of 9 (0 = no pain, 10 = worst possible pain).

9. _____ Denies pain c̄ Ⓡ UE movements.

10. _____ SLR is + on Ⓛ, − on Ⓡ.

11. _____ <u>Hx</u>: TIA in 1993, ASHD, CHF.

12. _____ Will be seen by PT 3 x/wk. as an O.P.

13. _____ Pt. will demonstrate indep gait s̄ device within 3 wks.

14. _____ Pt. states functional goal of returning to work in 3 wks.

15. _____ Will enquire if Pt. can be referred to OT & speech therapy.

16. _____ States hx of COPD since 1990.

17. _____ ↑ AROM Ⓡ shoulder to WNL within 2 mo. to allow Pt. to perform overhead work activities.

18. _____ Pt. became s.o.b. p̄ amb training c̄ a stair walker on 2 steps.

19. _____ Will resume PT on 1st day post-op per total knee care pathway.

20. _____ <u>Gait</u>: Indep c̄ crutches 50% PWB Ⓛ LE for 150 ft. x 2.

21. _____ Pt. was difficult to assess due to lack of cooperation as demonstrated by closing his eyes & crossing his arms when asked to stand.

22. _____ Unable to tolerate trunk flexion to sit for time periods functional for work situation (≈1 hr at a time s̄ standing).

Part II. Write the following information into clear, concise statements regarding treatment (include verbs to make the phrases/sentences complete).

1. Hot pack—20 minutes—twice per day—lumbar area

   Answer: _____

   _____

2. Ultrasound—7 minutes—1.0 watts per centimeter squared—right upper trapezius muscle—once per day.

   Answer: _____

   _____

3. Twice per day—progress patient through knee exercise program—attached

Answer: _____

_____

Part III. Read each of the following descriptions of treatment and state what is missing.

1. Pt. will receive Jobst pump Rx.

Answer: _____

_____

_____

2. Pt. will receive whirlpool c̄ Chlorazene BID.

Answer: _____

_____

_____

_____

_____

_____

Answer to "Writing Plan (P): Worksheet 1" are provided in Appendix A.

Writing Plan (P): WORKSHEET 2

Part I. Mark the statements that should be placed in the P category by placing a P on the blank line before each P statement. Also mark the Problem, S, O, and A statements by writing Prob, S, O, or A on the blank line before the appropriate statement.

1. _____ Biceps reflex 2+ Ⓡ, 3+ Ⓛ.

2. _____ Amb training, beginning in // bars & progressing to a walker.

3. _____ ↑ AROM Ⓛ knee to 0–115° within 2 wks. to allow Pt. to amb steps.

4. _____ C/o inability to use commode indep.

5. _____ Indep walker amb 150 x 2 50% PWB within 2 wks. to allow Pt. to amb around his home.

6. _____ Transfers: Supine ↔ sit c̄ max +1 assist.

7. _____ States was in a car accident & Pt.'s car was hit broadside on the passenger side.

8. _____ Pt. would like to return to her work as a secretary ASAP p̄ D/C.

9. _____ Pt. does not follow commands consistently, making much of the objective tests difficult to complete.

10. _____ Will be seen BID at B/S.

11. _____ C/o pain c̄ light touch of the scar on Ⓡ wrist.

12. _____ Sensation: Absent to light touch & pinprick throughout L5 distribution.

13. _____ C/o pain in "entire" Ⓛ LE c̄ active or passive movement of Ⓛ knee.

14. _____ Pt. will be given written & verbal instructions in home exercise & walking program.

15. _____ Indep in home exercise program of AROM Ⓡ LE within 2 wks.

16. _____ Proprioception: Min ↓ noted in entire Ⓛ LE.

17. _____ Will request an order for OT to assist c̄ dressing.

18. _____ Pt.'s nausea & vomiting during the past wk. have slowed progress of transfer training.

Part II. Write the following information into the P part of the note.

1. Sue Smith will be seen three times per week as an outpatient. You will first give her a pulsed ultrasound to her right shoulder at 1.5 W/cm² for 7 minutes. She'll then get mobilization to her right shoulder. You'll follow that up with an ice pack for 20 minutes. You also plan to teach her a home exercise program and attach a copy of it to your note. You also will ask her MD if she could be referred to OT for an ADL assessment since she states she cannot do anything for herself at home.

P: _____

_____

_____

_____

_____

_____

132

2. Rodney Racecar will receive treatment twice per day. He will be taught proper care of his residual limb and how to wrap his residual limb. He will receive resistive range of motion exercises to his legs beginning with 10 repetitions each and increasing the number of repetitions to tolerance. He will receive gait training with axillary crutches non-weight-bearing right leg and also transfer training.

P: _____

_____

_____

_____

_____

_____

Answers to "Writing Plan (P): Worksheet 2" are provided in Appendix A.

Review Worksheet: SOAP

Part I. Begin by turning to the corresponding answer sheet at the end of these instructions so that you can write your SOAP note directly on the answer sheet.

The following are the notes to yourself that you jotted down while reading the chart, interviewing the patient, and performing the objective tests. (While taking notes for yourself, you did not consult Hospital XYZ's approved abbreviations list nor were you particularly careful in your notation style.)

Write the information listed below into the Problem, *S*, and *O* portions of the note on the answer sheet. (Further instructions will be provided to help you write the *A* and *P* portions of the note.) Your note should be written to be an acceptable part of the patient's medical record at Hospital XYZ.

FROM THE CHART

Fractured right distal tibia and fractured right proximal humerus.
Patient has a cast applied to the tibia and is in a sling for the fractured humerus.

FROM THE SUBJECTIVE INTERVIEW

c/o pain in her right ankle while in a dependent position and severe pain in her right shoulder
    with elbow AAROM
Lives c̄ parents—1-story house—1 step at entrance—has carpeting throughout
Never used a wheelchair before
Patient is right handed
Is a high school student and wants to return to school ASAP p̄ D/C.
School is very academically challenging and competitive and does not believe she can stay out of
    school until she is healed.
School is on one level with no steps to enter the school. However, distances between classrooms
    are up to 1500 feet long. Has 7 class periods per day. All floor surfaces in school are linoleum.
Parents attended therapy with patient; state their insurance will rent the patient a wheelchair

FROM OBJECTIVE TESTS PERFORMED

Ⓛ UE—WNL AROM & strength
Ⓡ shoulder not assessed due to fracture
Ⓡ elbow AAROM is 30–70°
Ⓡ hand and wrist AROM very slow but WNL when patient is encouraged to complete full ROM
Ⓛ LE—WNL AROM & strength
Ⓡ LE—WNL at knee & hip—AROM
Ⓡ LE—strength N at knee & hip
Ⓡ LE—short leg cast Ⓡ ankle & foot so not assessed
Ⓡ LE—toes warm and normal color—able to wiggle toes
toilet transfers not assessed first visit
sit ↔ stand c̄ maximal +1 assist
supine ↔ sit c̄ moderate assistance of one person
W/c ↔ mat c̄ maximal +1 assist
NWB Ⓡ LE
NWB Ⓡ UE
Cried when Ⓡ ankle initially put in a dependent position
Unable to manage Ⓡ wheelchair brakes, or leg rest
Propelled wheelchair 10 feet using left leg and arm and was too exhausted to continue; required
    minimal assistance of 1 person and verbal cues to do so

Part II. In writing the assessment (*A*) and plan (*P*) portions of the note, follow these directions:

1. Under *A*, state that further assessment of the transfers not yet assessed (name them) is needed. Also comment that the patient should progress quickly in therapy but that the patient will need assistance with wheelchair propulsion at school at first until her endurance improves.

2. *Formulate a problem list* based on the *S* and *O* parts of the note.
   a. Look at the *S* portion of the note under *c/o*. Write this problem below.

   Problem: _____

   b. Look at the sections discussing the left extremities. Everything seems to be as normal as possible, considering the circumstances; therefore, it is not necessary to write anything about them in the problem list.

   c. Look at the sections discussing the right extremities. The LE seems to be as normal as possible in all areas except the ankle, and therapy cannot change the ankle at the current time; therefore, it is not necessary to write anything about the right lower extremity. Look at the elbow AAROM. Write the problem with the right elbow AAROM below.

   Problem: _____

   d. Look at the right hand and wrist AROM. They are at risk of losing full AROM. Write this as a problem below.

   Problem: _____

   e. Look at the transfer status. Write this problem below (remember that the problem list is a *summary*).

   Problem: _____

   f. Look at the patient's wheelchair management abilities. Write this problem below.

   Problem: _____

   g. Look at the patient's wheelchair propulsion abilities. Write this problem below.

   Problem: _____

Setting Priorities

Consider function first. Ambulation and wheelchair propulsion and management are the most functional problems. Write them as problem numbers 1, 2, and 3 on the answer sheet. (Transfers are needed in order to be able to use the wheelchair and should be the first priority. Wheelchair propulsion is not very possible or functional without the ability to manage the brakes and foot rests, so wheelchair management should be the second problem on the list.)

The patient's right elbow AAROM will definitely influence function if it is not resolved. This should be problem 4 on the list.

The patient's wrist and finger AAROM are in danger of decreasing. If they decrease, the patient's function will definitely decrease. This should be problem 5 on the list.

Although pain is a problem, the pain will naturally decrease with the passing of time when the ® LE is placed in and out of a dependent position during transfers. Therefore, this problem will not be considered to be of as much importance as the patient's functional problems. However, the problem is still of importance to the patient. Write this problem as problem number 6 on the answer sheet.

3. Using the information in the note, *set a long term goal for each problem*. (The problems are discussed individually below.)
   a. Requires assistance during transfers. You judge that the patient will be able to be independent and pain free in 10 days. (This combines problem numbers 1 and 6.) Write this as long term goal number 1 on the answer sheet.
   b. Requires assistance for wheelchair management. You judge that the patient will be able to be independent in 10 days. (Look at the note to make sure and include all of the types of surfaces on which the patient must ambulate.) Write this as long term goal number 2 on the answer sheet.

    c. Requires assistance for wheelchair propulsion. You judge that the patient will be able to be independent in 10 days and will be able to go about 100 feet. (Look at the note to make sure and include all of the types of surfaces on which the patient must propel her wheelchair.) Write this as long term goal number 3 on the answer sheet.

    d. Requires assistance with right elbow ROM and right elbow ROM is decreased. You judge that the patient will be independent in right elbow self-ROM exercises in 10 days. Write this as long term goal number four on the answer sheet. You also predict that the right elbow ROM will be at 15–90° in 10 days. Write this as long term goal number 5 on the answer sheet.

    e. The patient is at risk for decreased Ⓡ wrist and finger AROM. You judge that it will be full and pain free in 10 days. Write this as long term goal number 6 on the answer sheet.

4. *Set the short term goals* as follows:

    a. Consider the first long term goal *(transfers)*. Now look at the patient's present functional status (see the note). You first judge that the patient will be able to transfer sit ↔ stand and w/c ↔ mat with minimal assistance of 1 person in five days. Write this goal as number 1 on the answer sheet. You also estimate that the patient will be able to transfer supine ↔ sit with standby assistance of 1 person in five days. Write this goal as number 2 on the answer sheet.

       The transfers not yet assessed need to be assessed. This should be addressed in the *P* part of the note.

    b. Consider the second long term goal *(w/c management)*. Now look at the patient's present functional status (see the note). You judge that the patient should be able to manage her wheelchair brakes and leg rests with moderate assistance and verbal cues in five days. Write this goal as goal number 3 on the answer sheet.

    c. Consider the third long term goal *(wheelchair propulsion)*. You judge that the patient will be able to propel her wheelchair for about 50 feet with verbal cues only in five days. Write this goal as goal number 4 on the answer sheet.

5. Consider the fourth long term goal *(right elbow self-ROM exercises)*. You judge that the patient will require verbal cues only to perform right elbow self-ROM exercises in five days. Write this goal as goal number 5 on the answer sheet.

6. Consider the fifth long term goal *(right elbow ROM)*. You judge that the patient will have 25–80 degrees in five days. Write this goal as goal number 6 on the answer sheet.

7. Consider the sixth long term goal *(right wrist and finger AROM)*. You judge that the patient will be able to perform AROM exercises to right wrist and fingers independently in five days.

Write the treatment plan. Considering the short term goals, treatment must be planned to fulfill each goal. You decide to assess the transfers not yet assessed. You decide that you'll do transfer training (include all of the transfers that you want to teach the patient). You also decide that you will do training in wheelchair management and propulsion. You decide to perform ROM exercises (don't forget to list all of the joints involved, the type of ROM to each, and the exercises you plan to teach the patient). You will see the patient twice per day. Write this into the *P* portion of the note on the answer sheet.

Review Worksheet: SOAP Answer Sheet

Use this answer sheet to write the Problem, *S*, *O*, *A*, and *P* portions of a note according to the instructions given in the preceding pages. Use additional sheets of paper to complete your note as needed.

Problem List:

1. _____
2. _____
3. _____
4. _____
5. _____
6. _____
7. _____

Long Term Goals:

1. _____
   _____
2. _____
   _____
3. _____
   _____
4. _____
5. _____
   _____
6. _____
   _____

Short Term Goals:

1. _____
   _____
   _____
2. _____
   _____
3. _____
4. _____
   _____
5. _____
   _____
   _____
6. _____
7. _____
   _____
8. _____
   _____

P: _____

_____

_____

_____

_____

_____

_____

_____

_____

_____

_____

Use this answer sheet to write the Problem, *S*, *O*, *A*, and *P* portions of a functional outcomes note using the same information as in the note above. Use additional sheets of paper to complete your note as needed. Hint: The number of blanks left for the Problem List, Long Term Goals, and Short Term Goals may be more than should be needed for a functional outcomes note.

_____

_____

_____

_____

_____

_____

_____

_____

_____

_____

_____

_____

_____

_____

_____

_____

_____

_____

_____

140

Problem List:

1. _____

2. _____

3. _____

4. _____

5. _____

6. _____

7. _____

Expected Functional Outcomes:

1. _____
   _____

2. _____
   _____

3. _____
   _____

4. _____

5. _____
   _____

6. _____
   _____

Short Term Goals:

1. _____
   _____
   _____

2. _____
   _____

3. _____

4. _____
   _____

5. _____
   _____
   _____

6. _____

7. _____
   _____

8. _____
   _____

P: _____

_____

_____

_____

_____

_____

_____

_____

_____

_____

_____

Answers to "Review Worksheet: SOAP" are provided in Appendix A.

13 Various Applications of SOAP

This workbook has covered the reasons for writing notes and a brief history of the origins of the SOAP note (the POMR). It has offered a test of your working knowledge of medical terminology and a good review of abbreviations.

Applying SOAP to Other Note Formats

As you begin to practice in clinical settings, you will find that nobody writes notes exactly as you were taught to write notes. Each facility that uses the SOAP format has its own variations of the format. Within any facility using the SOAP note format, each therapist has his or her own variations of the format.

Many facilities do not use a SOAP note format at all. Some facilities use a single narrative style format. Others use an outline format of some kind. Still others (especially private practice settings) may send letters to the patient's physician describing the patient's condition, goals, plans, and so forth. School settings and/or chronic care settings may set yearly goals as part of a student's or patient's individual education plan (IEP). Some facilities are moving toward various types of functional outcomes reports. Whatever the format that you may encounter, your knowledge of writing SOAP notes should be helpful.

Narrative notes frequently include the same information used in the SOAP note format, but the information may be in a different order and is not labeled SOAP

Outline note formats, or *fill-in-the-blank forms,* also include the information that a SOAP note contains. The information may be organized in a different order, and periods and/or sentences may not be used, but the information is still present. As long as you know how to organize the information and put the information into the categories used in the SOAP note, you will only need to learn where to put the *S* information or the *O* information or the goals or treatment plan in an unfamiliar format or form.

Letters written to a physician's office on a regular basis are also usually organized in a particular style in order to save time. Certain categories are placed in a certain order, according to the standards set forth by the physical therapy practice involved. If you know your **143** SOAP categories, you will be able to rearrange them to fit into a letter format.

Individual educational programs (IEPs) also have a standardized format that takes the information involved in a SOAP note and renames and rearranges the categories. Goals that are set yearly become the long term goals. Whether they are officially written or not, short term goals to be achieved by different times during the year are set in order to meet the long term goals. The goal format taught in this workbook is very adequate for use in most educational settings.

Functional outcomes reporting is still very new in the health professions and varies from some sort of adaptation of the SOAP format to a report format that is organized very differently from the SOAP format. Remember that a functional outcomes reporting format usually includes *only* information that relates to function.

Finally, not every facility that writes SOAP notes includes every part of the SOAP note covered in this workbook. Certain facilities do not include the problem list. Others combine the *A* and *P* portions of the note and list each problem, its corresponding long term goal, short term goal(s), and treatment together before moving on the next problem. There are as many variations on the SOAP note as there are facilities that use the SOAP note format.

Uses in Problem Solving

One of the reasons that the SOAP note format is so adaptable to other styles of note writing is that SOAP is more than a type of note format. **SOAP is a method of identifying, working through, and solving the patient's problems.** Although you were not expected to independently identify the problems, set goals, or generate treatment programs in this workbook, you were given many examples of how the SOAP note format can be used to plan a patient's care. As long as you use the SOAP format for yourself in approaching and solving patient problems, you can learn to write the information in any form that you might like. A comparison of the problem-solving process and use of the SOAP note is included in Appendix B of this workbook.

A Word to the PTA or COTA

Many of the examples in this workbook included writing an entire initial evaluation. According to the standards of the professions, PTAs and COTAs usually do not write initial notes. However, the skills that you used to write the initial and discharge notes in this workbook can be used in writing interim notes in your daily practice. Many facilities ask the assistant to write the interim note and to document the goals and treatment set by the therapist and assistant together for their patients. One of the ways in which you can be most helpful to the therapists with whom you work is to assist them with the documentation included in patient care. Therefore, it is important that your skills in this area continue to be used and improved long after you no longer need this workbook.

Documenting All Types of Patient Care

Most of the cases used in this workbook were quite simple. Some of your instructors may disagree with the method of documenting the details of the cases listed within this workbook. (Example: There are quite a few acceptable methods of documenting AROM.) As you approach learning while in school and throughout your career, be aware of the methods available to document what you learn, no matter what the subject matter. Ask your instructors how they document the information that they are teaching you. Ask for definitions of terminology such as "minimal," "moderate," and "maximal" as you begin to practice in various clinical facilities. Be aware of articles that you read that may define and describe terminology for you as they discuss evaluation techniques and scales.

As professions, physical and occupational therapy still have much to do to standardize terminology used in documentation. Many facilities do not have written definitions for commonly used terms, such as physical assistance given or balance. The methods used to describe the evaluation results of all types of patients vary widely throughout the country.

While the variations in descriptive terminology demonstrate the wide number of approaches and techniques available to therapists, the allied health professions desperately need to work to standardize some of the terminology used in order to be understood by other professionals, third-party readers, and each other. *Physical Therapy, American Journal of Occupational Therapy,* and other medical and rehabilitation journals contain many articles discussing evaluation and rating scales for patients with various diagnoses and conditions. Each individual clinical facility adopting and using some of the scales already developed and validated will begin the large task of standardization that faces the allied health professions.

Your experience in writing notes and documenting what you do as a therapist has barely begun with the completion of this workbook. You have learned to write SOAP notes, to organize the information into categories within each section of the note, to be clear and concise in what you say, and to use abbreviations and medical terminology well. The application of the information is now up to you.

As with any skill, the continued use and practice of note writing will perfect your skills. You will adapt all that you have learned about writing notes to the style of each facility in which you practice. Eventually, even if you practice in a facility with a particular note-writing style, you will develop a style that is unique to you. You can develop expertise in documentation and help move the profession toward more standardized methods of evaluation and documentation.

In the immediate future, you may wish to remove the appendices from this workbook and keep them available as quick references on documentation. They summarize some of the information included in this workbook. They can assist you in applying what you have learned about writing notes as you continue the process of developing yourself as a member of the healthcare team.

Moving into the 14 Future: Documentation Forms, Medicare Forms, and Computerized Documentation

What will the future hold for documentation by rehabilitation professionals and other medical professionals? As trends in health care change, documentation will change. Healthcare professionals are constantly looking for a more efficient and effective way to ease the task of documentation without losing their ability to act as professionals. Therefore, systems of documentation that can be performed at the point of care have been developed at some facilities and are currently being developed by other healthcare facilities and outside companies. In the meantime, Medicare has developed Forms 700 and 701 for purposes of obtaining consistent data that can assist Medicare reviewers with the determination of the appropriateness of the care given to the patients.

Well-written SOAP notes, documentation forms, Medicare forms, and computerized documentation share one characteristic: they provide structure to documentation. Structured documentation guarantees the collection of a consistent data set that can give us information about the outcomes and effectiveness of the treatment that we give our patients. Without this type of information, we will not be able to meet the challenges of managing both the cost and the quality of healthcare delivery.

Medicare Forms

Medicare has developed Forms 700, 701, and 702 in an attempt to gather consistent data needed to make decisions about whether the patient's condition and treatment qualifies for Medicare coverage. Before these forms were developed, reviewers for Medicare were receiving poor quality patient notes, some without goals, some without a good description of the patient's functional problems. If you look at the Medicare forms, they ask for (1) demographic data (the patient's name, age, and Social Security or Medicare number), (2) basic medical data (date of surgery or onset of condition, diagnosis), and (3) data that should already be contained in a well-written SOAP note. The data they request include functional status prior to treatment and current functional status, long term goals and short term goals (short term goals are listed as monthly goals), treatment plan, and justification for treatment. It is easy to include the information required by these forms since the categories are the same as those of any good SOAP note.

Documentation Forms and Computerized Documentation Programs

In some facilities, forms are used for documentation or documentation is done on the computer. Each facility usually has its unique documentation forms or type of computerized documentation format. The purpose of this section is to review some advantages and disadvantages of each of these formats for documentation and to include items for consideration when developing forms or looking to purchase a computerized documentation system.

DOCUMENTATION FORMS

Documentation forms are used in many clinics for many reasons. Some of the reasons include the following:

- Decreasing the amount of writing by the therapist/assistant
- Increasing the efficiency of the therapist/assistant in documenting patient care
- Increasing the consistency of documentation (and thus fulfilling certain quality assurance or legal/risk management requirements) by building certain components into a note, such as whether the patient is given a home program and his or her level of independence in performing the home program
- Making the data gathered for outcomes studies more consistent
- Making functional information easier to read by all parties who use the information

Forms are usually individualized to fit the needs of the individual healthcare institution and its patient population. When designing a form, a good place to start is by watching clinicians practice. Forms should include the items commonly assessed by the therapist. Other additions to the forms can be obtained by asking staff members to use the forms and give feedback to those designing the forms.

When beginning to use a new form, it is important for the therapist/assistant to give himself or herself time to adapt to the use of the form. Becoming familiar with a form before seeing a patient makes the therapist much more efficient in the use of the form.

The most efficient use of a form is to complete the form, or at least begin its completion, while seeing the patient. If you can write your subjective and objective findings directly on the form, you will save time. *Caution:* Do not let the use of forms limit your practice! If an item is missing from a form, find a place to write it (if it is relevant to the patient's function). Also, forms should be revised on a regular basis to meet the needs of good clinical practice.

TYPES OF DOCUMENTATION FORMS. Several types of documentation forms are in use in various facilities. These include the following:

- Flow sheets (see Appendix F for an example of types/uses of flow sheets).
- Initial assessment/discharge note forms.

- Interim/discharge note forms.
- One-visit-only documentation forms.
- Supplement forms to be attached to initial, interim, or discharge forms. These forms often have specialized tests or scales that are only needed with certain types of patients.

DEVELOPMENT OF DOCUMENTATION FORMS. When developing a form, the following should be considered:

- Don't reinvent the wheel unless you really must. Revising a form from another facility (used with permission, of course) is much easier than starting with nothing.
- When you have developed a draft version of the form, ask yourself and those who must use and read the forms if the form does what it is supposed to do for all parties involved (healthcare providers, those concerned with reimbursement, etc.).
- Communicate with all parties involved when you develop forms. If the form is to be useful, everyone must know how to use the form (both writing on the form and reading the form).
- Subjective and objective items frequently assessed by the staff should be included.
- If a standard scale, test, or definition of measurement is used by all staff to measure or document a certain characteristic of the patient or a certain facet of patient care, a checklist may be faster in documenting the care.
- Checklists can save therapist time and add speed in documentation.
- If you use any sort of checklists in your note forms, try to make the checklists consistent or similar from one form to another. This saves confusion and unnecessary staff reorientation time.
- Frequently leave space for very brief comments or descriptions.
- Unless the form is created with a very specific patient population in mind, allow for a general assessment of the patient.
- If there are no standardized methods of documenting the information derived from your assessment of the patient, allow room for writing.
- Forms will influence practice, so make sure to include items that you believe are essential to practice.
- If the staff has been writing SOAP notes, transition for the staff will be easier if you follow a SOAP format. Because SOAP is a problem-solving format, documenting using this format on a form assists the staff in problem solving.
- Function should still be stated first in the subjective and objective portions of the note form, just as you should do so when writing a SOAP note.

COMPUTERIZED DOCUMENTATION

Computerized documentation is still in the stages of development. Some facilities have a well-developed program that is tailored to the needs of that facility. Within the next few years, many improvements will be seen in the area of computerized documentation. This section will serve as a review of some of the features that have been developed or are in stages of development by various companies throughout the country.

The advantage of computerized documentation over the use of forms is that the limitations of paper (trying to get all the necessary information into a limited amount of space) become unimportant since the computer is not limited to any particular size in which to place the information gathered. Computers can also have all of the possible tests and measurements available, so the therapist is not limited by the tests and measurements available on a given form.

Some features that have been developed or are in stages of development that will make computers even easier to use in the future are the following:

- *Data can be entered by making choices and simply touching a stylus to the screen.* This makes data entry more consistent and does not require keyboard competence.
- *Data can be printed in a variety of formats.* The Medicare Forms 700 and 701 no longer require extra time because the information can be printed in the form of a Form 700 or 701 for reimbursement purposes and in the form of a SOAP note for the medical record. It could

also allow the therapist to choose certain functional or relevant data to send to the patient's physician or other referral source. This technology will be ready very soon.

- *The medical record can be retrieved and notes written at the patient's bedside.* Some healthcare facilities have computers located in every patient's room or between every two rooms. With notebook computer technology available, the therapist will be able to have a notebook with him or her that contains and/or can access the patient's medical record and rehab information for all the patients the therapist treats.

- *All documentation can be completed at bedside.* Even outpatient and home healthcare therapists will be able to have the computer with them and complete all documentation while they work with the patient. Notebook computers with removable keyboards are already available. Modems make retrieval of the patient's medical record possible. Development in this area will be completed soon.

- *Handwriting recognition is a feature that will be developed more in the next few years.* This will enable the therapist to enter extra notes and information as needed (much as therapists now do when they use forms and need to remark about the unusual quality of a movement).

- *Voice recognition is a feature that will also be developed more in the next few years.* This could completely change our methods of data entry, although some caution must be taken in the use of voice-activated methodology while at the patient's bedside.

- *Charging will be able to be done by the therapist immediately upon completing the patient's treatment and while he or she completes other computerized documentation (and the computer may remind the therapist to charge the patient).* Computerized charging systems exist in many clinics today. Moving the charging to the patient's bedside, along with all other documentation functions, will greatly increase therapist efficiency and relieve the repetition in documentation that some therapists experience today.

When looking at computerized documentation systems, items that deserve consideration are listed below.

- It is important to consider the needs of therapists at their individual practice sites. A system should be flexible enough to fulfill the needs of the therapist at the individual practice site; otherwise, the system is not worthwhile.

- Computerized documentation systems vary in their mobility, weight, flexibility, ease of use, speed of data entry, and speed of the hardware. All of these factors must be considered when purchasing or developing a computerized system.

- Training time must be taken into consideration when you discuss the cost of a computerized documentation system. A system that requires extensive training must also save much time in order to be cost effective.

- Technology is only worthwhile if it makes the therapist's task of documentation easier and allows him or her to do something he or she could not do without the technology. For example, the time spent documenting should be decreased, and spelling errors or obvious errors in the recording of data should be pointed out to the therapist automatically for the purpose of immediate correction.

- The willingness, availability, and cost of programmers to customize the system to the individual facility's needs should be investigated before making a commitment to a computerized documentation system.

Summary

Many facilities have found the development of documentation forms helpful in assisting therapists to document faster and more efficiently. Forms must be developed by a facility's therapists to meet their practice needs.

Computerized documentation will definitely be the mode of documentation in the future. Just as documentation forms must be customized to the practice at an individual practice site, computerized programs must be customized to meet the needs of therapists at an individual site.

Forms and computerized documentation do not exclude the type of thinking that is used in SOAP note writing. As mentioned in Chapter 13, the SOAP note format assists therapists in structuring their thinking about patient problems and the attainment of the patient's goals for function. As forms and computer programs are further developed, aspects of the SOAP problem-solving format will continue to be used to assist the therapist in meeting patient needs while he or she documents.

Answers to Worksheets

The answers to the worksheets are on the following pages. In order to get the most benefit from these answer sheets, it is suggested that you refer to them only *after* you have completed the worksheets. Their purpose is to serve as a means to check your work and to learn.

CHAPTER 3: Using Abbreviations

WORKSHEET 1

Part I

1. To physical therapy by wheelchair
   Turn the patient every hour
2. The diagnosis is rheumatoid arthritis; rule out systemic lupus erythematosus.
3. Rx: OD, ADL training, US @ 1.0–1.5 W/cm² to ant. superior Ⓡ knee for 5 min.
4. The patient complains of shortness of breath after bilateral upper extremity proprioceptive neuromuscular facilitation exercises.
5. The patient's diagnosis is multiple sclerosis; rule out organic brain syndrome.
6. Pt. is a BK amputee c̄ a PTB prosthesis c̄ a SACH foot.
7. Pt.'s HR ↑ 20 bpm p̄ 2 min. of self-care ADLs.
8. Pt. amb in // bars FWB Ⓛ LE for ~20 ft. x 2 c̄ min assist. of 1 person (or c̄ +1 min assist. or c̄ min +1 assist.)

9. UE strength is N throughout bilat.
10. <u>Short term goal</u>: ↓ dependence in transfers w/c → bed to mod assist. within 1 wk.

CHAPTER 3: Using Abbreviations

WORKSHEET 2

Part I

1. The patient complains of right hip pain after ambulating approximately 300 feet once with a walker full weight bearing on the right lower extremity.
2. Pt. may be 50% PWB Ⓛ LE.
   v.o. Dr. Smith/your signature, PT or OTR
3. Discontinue ultrasound in the area of the right sacroiliac joint.
4. The diagnosis is fractured left clavicle and subluxation of the left sternoclavicular joint.
5. The patient's fasting blood sugar upon admission was over 300.
6. <u>Dx</u>: Ⓛ CVA.
7. Muscle function test: G strength throughout UEs bilat.
8. X-ray reveals fx Ⓛ 3rd metacarpal immediately proximal to the MCP joint.
9. To OT for ADL.
   v.o. Dr. Jones/your signature, PT or OTR
10. The physician's impression is that the patient has a peripheral neuropathy; rule out central nervous system dysfunction.

CHAPTER 4: Medical Terminology

WORKSHEET 1

Part I

1. Osteoma
2. Hypoglycemia
3. Subcutaneous
4. Suprapubic
5. Dorsal/posterior
6. Cephalad
7. Erythema
8. Intercostal
9. Anterior or ventral
10. Afferent

Part II

1. Fusion of the pubic bones medially (growth of the bones together)
2. Enlargement of the heart
3. Removal of a meniscus
4. Cartilaginous tumor
5. Fusion of a joint
6. Surgical opening of the skull
7. The study of the nervous system
8. Without sensation
9. Inflammation of a vein
10. Abnormally high blood pressure

CHAPTER 4: Medical Terminology

WORKSHEET 2

Part I

1. Arthritis
2. Arthroscopy
3. Myopathy
4. Dyspnea
5. Ataxia
6. Chondromalacia
7. Encephalitis
8. Meningioma
9. Hemiplegia
10. Subclavicular

Part II

1. Without pain
2. Affecting both sides
3. Opposite side
4. Lack of speech
5. Inflammation of a tendon
6. Slowness of movement
7. Difficulty swallowing
8. Pain in the joints
9. Softening of the brain
10. Pertaining to a rib and its cartilage

CHAPTER 6: Writing Subjective (S)

WORKSHEET 1 (ALSO INCLUDED: STATING THE PROBLEM)

Part I

1. S
2.
3. This is *not* S because objective testing is required to ascertain whether the motion reproduces the pain.
4.
5.
6. S
7.
8.
9. S
10. Prob.
11.
12.
13.
14. S
15.
16. Prob.
17.
18.
19.
20. S
21.
22. S

Part II

1. Dx: ℝ shoulder bursitis.
2. Dx: Ⓛ shoulder subluxation. s/p ℝ CVA 1 yr.
3. Dx: Resp. failure. Hx: COPD & CHF.

Part III

A. 1, 4, 6, 5
B. 7
C. 3
D. 9
E. 2, 8 (8, 2 is also acceptable)

Part IV

1. a. Hx:
   b. States fell at home.
   c. (1) When did the patient fall?
      (2) How did the patient fall?
      (3) What was the patient doing when she fell?
2. a. Hx:
   b. States onset of pain in the p.m. of [date].
3. a. c/o:
   b. c/o min pain ℝ foot on this date.
   c. (1) The exact location of the pain in the ℝ foot.
      (2) Rating the pain on a pain scale.
4. a. Home situation:
   b. States lives alone. Describes 2 steps c̄ handrail on ℝ ascending at the entrance of her home.

5. a. Pain behavior:
   b. States pain is located from ℝ hand through the ℝ forearm on this date. Pain limits typing to 5 min. at a time.

Part V

1. <u>Problem</u>: 58 y/o ♂ c̄ dx of minor ligamentous injury ℝ knee or <u>Dx</u>: Minor ligamentous injury ℝ knee.
   S: <u>Present c/o</u>: ℝ knee pain which Pt. describes as constant & "burning." Rates pain intensity as 7 (0 = no pain, 10 = worst possible pain). Pain is ↓ c̄ rest & ↑ c̄ walking. Denies pain during ℝ knee flexion. <u>Hx</u>: States fell at work landing on ℝ knee 1st. <u>Home situation</u>: States lives c̄ wife in 2nd-floor apartment. Describes 9 steps c̄ handrail Ⓛ ascending to access apartment c̄ no elevator available. <u>Lifestyle/goals</u>: States is a carpenter. Short term goal: To access his apartment indep. Long term goal: To resume former busy lifestyle, including return to work.

2. **S**: <u>c/o</u>: pain, swelling, & stiffness Ⓛ hand & wrist. Pain ↓ c̄ rest & ↑ c̄ grasping or wt.-bearing activities Ⓛ UE. Describes pain of an intensity of 5 (0 = no pain, 10 = worst possible pain) c̄ typing. Swelling & stiffness occur when Pt. tries to move Ⓛ hand & wrist; swelling is worse p̄ work.
   <u>Hx</u>: Fell at work & landed on Ⓛ hand c̄ wrist extended. Denies previous injuries or previous use of splint Ⓛ UE.
   <u>Home situation</u>: Lives c̄ wife; will not have to cook or lift heavy objects at home until ready.
   <u>Functional limitations</u>: Occupation as transcriptionist; types up to 8 hrs./day; physician told Pt. to limit typing to 4 hrs./day until edema stops. Having difficulty eating s̄ use of ℝ hand (is Ⓛ-hand dominant).
   <u>Pt. goals</u>: To return to former lifestyle, including typing at work (long term). To hold a fork s̄ pain (short term).

CHAPTER 6: Writing Subjective (*S*)

WORKSHEET 2 (ALSO INCLUDED: STATING THE PROBLEM)

Part I

A. 8
B. 1, 5, 7 (numbers could be interchanged)
C. 3, 4
D. 9, 2 (9 was placed before 2; 2 further explains 9)
E. 6

Part II

1. a. c/o
   b. C/o pain ℝ LE proximal to the knee.
   c. (1) Exact location of the pain is still unclear. Is the pain in the anterior or posterior portion of the ℝ LE proximal to the knee? (2) Putting the pain on a pain scale would have been helpful.

2. a. Prior level of function/Pt. goals:
   b. States depended on his wife to bathe him prior to his CVA. Plans to cont. to depend on wife for bathing p̄ D/C.

3. a. c/o
   b. States cannot dress herself.

4. a. Prior level of function: or Hx:
   b. Denies use of a walker PTA.

Part III

1.
2.
3.
4. *S*
5.
6.
7. *S*
8.
9.
10. Prob.
11. *S*
12.
13.
14.
15. *S*
16.
17.
18.
19. *S*

Part IV

<u>Dx</u>: Contusion Ⓛ hip.
S: <u>c/o</u>: Ⓛ hip pain of intensity of 8 (0 = no pain, 10 = worst possible pain) when FWB Ⓛ LE. Denies Ⓛ hip pain while sitting or supine. <u>Hx</u>: States fell in kitchen on Ⓛ hip in a.m. of (date); was able to get up s̄ help; experienced pain throughout the day. Pt. went to ER in late p.m. of same date. Used a walker p̄ Ⓛ THR in 1990. <u>Home status</u>: Lives alone in an apartment. Apartment building has elevator & only elevations Pt. needs to amb are curbs. <u>Prior level of function</u>: Amb indep s̄ device immediately PTA & was indep in all ADLs. <u>Current functional level</u>: Spends time in a w/c rented by the family. <u>Pt. goals</u>: Indep ADLs c̄ walker.

CHAPTER 7: Writing Objective (*O*)

WORKSHEET 1

Part I

1.
2. *O*
3.
4. *S*

5. O
6. S
7.
8. S
9. Prob.
10. O
11.
12. S
13.
14. O
15.
16.
17.
18. O
19. O
20.
21. S
22.

Part II

1. D
2. E
3. D
4. A
5. E
6. C
7. A
8. B
9. A
10. E
11. B

Part III

1. a. <u>Strength</u>:
   b. G in bilat. UEs.
2. a. <u>Trunk</u>:
   b. SLR Ⓛ reproduces Pt.'s worst back pain.
3. a. <u>Strength</u>:
   b. N Ⓡ shoulder musculature, G Ⓡ biceps, P Ⓡ triceps, O all Ⓡ UE musculature distal to the elbow. Ⓛ UE strength is N. **or** <u>Strength</u>: Ⓡ UE: N shoulder musculature, G biceps, P triceps, O all musculature distal to the elbow. Ⓛ UE: N throughout.
4. a. <u>Amb</u>:
   b. Indep for ~150 ft. x 2 FWB c̄ walker.
5. a. <u>Endurance</u>:
   b. Pt. was SOB p̄ transferring supine → sit & bed → B/S chair; resp. rate ↑ from 18 resp./min. ā the transfers to 32 resp./min. immediately p̄ the transfers.
6. a. <u>AROM</u>: **or** Ⓛ LE:
   b. <u>AROM</u>: Ⓛ ankle WNL. **or** Ⓛ LE: Ankle AROM WNL.

Part IV

1. <u>UEs</u>: Strength & AROMs WNL.
2. <u>Amb</u>: Indep c̄ walker NWB Ⓛ LE 150 ft. x 2
3. Ⓛ LE: Long leg cast.
4. Ⓡ LE: AROM & strength WNL.
5. <u>Transfers</u>: On/off toilet c̄ min +1 assist. (**or** c̄ +1 min assist. **or** c̄ min assist. of 1), sit ↔ stand &

supine ↔ sit (**or** supine ↔ sit & sit ↔ stand) indep.
6. <u>Amb</u>: ↑ & ↓ 1 step c̄ a walker c̄ min +1 assist. (**or** c̄ +1 min assist. **or** c̄ min assist. of 1).
7. <u>Amb</u>: c̄ walker in & out of a door, including opening/closing door, c̄ min +1 assist. (**or** c̄ +1 min assist. **or** c̄ min assist. of 1).
   or <u>Amb</u>: Opens/closes & amb through a door c̄ walker c̄ min +1 assist.
8. Ⓛ LE: Not further assessed.

Part V

A. 2, 7†, 6†
B. 5
C. 1*, 4*
D. 3, 8

*1 & 4 were put in that order because of the order of the heading.
†7 & 6 are interchangeable; 7 was placed first because walking in and out of a door occurs more frequently during daily life than ambulating 1 step.

Part VI

O: <u>Amb</u>: c̄ walker indep NWB Ⓛ LE 150 ft. x 2 on level surfaces. Requires min +1 assist. to open/close door & to amb in/out of door c̄ walker. 1-step elevation c̄ walker c̄ min +1 assist.
<u>Transfers</u>: Min. +1 on/off toilet, indep. sit ↔ stand & supine ↔ sit. <u>UEs</u> & Ⓡ LE: Strength & AROMs WNL throughout. Ⓛ LE: Long leg cast; not further assessed.

(Variations similar to those discussed after each statement are acceptable.)

CHAPTER 7: Writing Objective (*O*)

WORKSHEET 2

Parts I and II

1. O   Impair
2. S   (Impair is acceptable if you believe a statement of history helps you understand the impairment better. It is *not* a functional statement.)
3.
4.
5.
6.
7. S   Func
8. O   Func
9. Prob.
10.
11. O   Impair
12. S   Impair
13. O   Impair
14.
15.

16. *O* Impair
17.
18. *S* Impair

Parts III and IV

1. D Impair
2. B Func
3. E Impair
4. E or F Impair
5. D Impair
6. E Impair
7. F Impair
8. C Impair
9. E Impair
10. E Impair
11. A Func
12. D Impair
13. E Impair
14. B Func
15. D Impair
16. E Impair

Part V

_____ UEs
_____ LEs
_____ trunk
___X___ transfers
___X___ amb
_____ Rx
___X___ endurance (Use of the category called "endurance" is optional because the information could be placed under the "ambulation" category.)
___X___ strength
___X___ AROM
_____ ℝ extremities
_____ ADL
_____ Ⓛ extremities

Because the strength of *both* UEs and LEs is the same and *almost* all ROM is WNL bilaterally, it is most efficient to categorize according to tests performed (versus parts of the body tested).

Part VI

A. 2, 6 (You could have decided to use an endurance category and placed this under "Endurance.")
B. 1
C. 3, 4
D. 5
E. 6 (if you decided not to use the statement in A above)

Part VII

O: <u>Amb</u>: Stood FWB in // bars 1 min. x 2 then took 1 step c̄ min +1 assist. Fatigued p̄ standing x 2; all other assessment deferred. <u>Transfers</u>: Sit ↔ stand c̄ min +1 assist. <u>AROM</u>: All WNL UEs & LEs except ~90° shoulder abduction & ~100° shoulder flexion bilat. <u>Strength</u>: LE & UE strength at least F (group muscle assessment performed); unable to further assess due to mental status.

Note: The categories of strength and AROM could be written with either category listed first.

CHAPTER 7: Writing Objective (*O*)

WORKSHEET 3

Part I

a. 6
b. 1
c. 2
d. 7, 3, 4, 5

Note: The sections of the note could be in a different order but should be arranged somewhat logically, and the statements within the sections should be in logical order.

Part II

O: <u>Transfers</u>: Supine ↔ sit c̄ mod +1 assist. for ℝ LE movement. W/c ↔ mat c̄ sliding board c̄ max +1 assist. to place sliding board & remove w/c armrest; min +1 assist. during actual transfer to assist c̄ NWB status ℝ LE; verbal cues for hand placement. <u>W/c mobility</u>: Propels forward indep. 15 ft. x 2; requires assist. to maneuver w/c close to mat & lock brakes. <u>Endurance</u>: Requires frequent rest periods during Rx. <u>LE strength</u>: Hip flexors G Ⓛ, G− ℝ; hip abductors at least F bilat. but not assessed against gravity. Knee flexors G Ⓛ. <u>Rx this date</u> (or any other simple title): Bilat. hip abduction/adduction c̄ 2# (supine) & SLR x 15; Ⓛ knee flex & terminal ext. c̄ 2# x 15. Transfer & w/c mobility & management training.

Part III

O: FUNCTIONAL LIMITATIONS: <u>Transfers</u>: Supine ↔ sit c̄ mod +1 assist. for ℝ LE movement. W/c ↔ mat c̄ sliding board c̄ max +1 assist. to place sliding board & remove w/c armrest; min +1 assist. during actual transfer to asset. c̄ NWB status ℝ LE; verbal cues for hand placement. <u>W/c mobility</u>: Propels forward indep 15 ft. x 2; requires assist. to maneuver w/c close to mat & lock brakes. <u>Reaction to Rx this date</u>: Tolerated bilat. hip abduction/adduction c̄ 2# (supine) & SLR x 15, & Ⓛ knee flex & terminal ext c̄ 2# x 15. Received transfer & w/c mobility & management training. Requires frequent rest periods during Rx.

PHYSICAL IMPAIRMENTS: <u>LE strength</u>: Hip flexors G Ⓛ, G− ℝ; hip abductors at least F bilat. but not assessed against gravity. Knee flexors G Ⓛ.

Part IV

1. a. <u>Amb</u>:
   b. Pt. amb. 50 ft. x 2 c̄ 50% PWB Ⓛ LE c̄ standby assist. due to vision deficits.

2. a. $\underline{\textcircled{L} \text{ LE}}$:
   b. 2+ pitting edema $\textcircled{L}$ ankle.
3. a. $\underline{\text{LEs}}$:
   b. KJ: 3+ $\textcircled{R}$, 2+ $\textcircled{L}$.
4. a. $\underline{\text{Transfers}}$:
   b. Pt. transfers w/c $\leftrightarrow$ mat $\bar{c}$ sliding board $\bar{c}$ standby assist. +1 (**or** standby +1 assist. **or** standby assist. of 1) for balance.
5. a. $\underline{\text{Bed mobility}}$: **or** $\underline{\text{Rolling}}$: **or** $\underline{\text{ADLs}}$:
   b. Rolls supine $\rightarrow$ sidelying $\textcircled{L}$ or $\textcircled{R}$ $\bar{c}$ max. +2 assist. (**or** +2 max assist. **or** max assist. of 2).

CHAPTER 7: Writing Objective (*O*)

WORKSHEET 4

Part I

a. 3, 7
b. 1, 2, 4, 5
c. 6

Part II

There are probably many correct ways to organize this information. This student did a nice job organizing the information above. Another way to organize it would be to use the following categories: $\underline{\text{Amb}}$, $\underline{\text{Transfers}}$, $\textcircled{R}$ UE, $\textcircled{L}$ UE & LEs. This method would allow the reader to see that the $\textcircled{L}$ UE and LEs are relatively normal and then to get an accurate view of the $\textcircled{R}$ UE.

O: $\underline{\text{Amb}}$: $\bar{c}$ walker $\bar{c}$ min +1 assist. for 50 ft. x 1 wt. bearing as tolerated all extremities. $\underline{\text{Transfers}}$: W/c $\leftrightarrow$ mat pivot $\bar{c}$ min +1 assist. (**or** +1 min. assist. **or** $\bar{c}$ min. assist. of 1), sit $\leftrightarrow$ supine indep. $\textcircled{R}$ UE: *Appearance:* Incision $\textcircled{R}$ ant. forearm covered $\bar{c}$ steristrips. *AROM:* Limited shoulder flex. to ~120°, abd. to ~70°; elbow flex. WNL, ext. −42°; wrist flex. WNL, ext. to neutral $\bar{c}$ full finger flex. *Strength:* $\textcircled{R}$ shoulder flexors F+; elbow flexors & extensors, wrist flexors & extensors, finger flexors & extensors G. *Sensation:* To light touch & sharp/dull WNL. $\textcircled{L}$ UE & LEs: *AROM:* WNL throughout. *Strength* (gross break test used): N throughout $\textcircled{L}$ UE & $\textcircled{R}$ LE. $\textcircled{L}$ LE G all muscle groups. *Sensation:* To light touch & sharp/dull WNL throughout.

Part III

O: FUNCTIONAL LIMITATIONS: $\underline{\text{Amb}}$: $\bar{c}$ walker $\bar{c}$ min +1 assist. for 50 ft. x 1 wt. bearing as tolerated all extremities. $\underline{\text{Transfers}}$: W/c $\leftrightarrow$ mat pivot $\bar{c}$ min +1 assist. (**or** +1 min. assist. **or** $\bar{c}$ min. assist. of 1), sit $\leftrightarrow$ supine indep.
PHYSICAL IMPAIRMENTS: $\textcircled{R}$ UE: *Appearance:* Incision $\textcircled{R}$ ant. forearm covered $\bar{c}$ steristrips. *AROM:* Limited shoulder flex. to ~120°, abd. to

~70°; elbow flexion WNL, extension −42°; wrist flexion WNL, extension to neutral $\bar{c}$ full finger flexion. *Strength:* $\textcircled{R}$ shoulder flexors F+; elbow flexors & extensors, wrist flexors & extensors, finger flexors & extensors G. $\textcircled{L}$ UE & LEs: *Strength* (gross break test used): $\textcircled{L}$ LE G all muscle groups.

REVIEW WORKSHEET: STATING THE PROBLEM, *S* AND *O*

Part I

1. *O*
2.
3.
4. *S*
5. *O*
6. Prob.
7. *S*
8. *S*
9.
10. Prob.
11. *O*
12. *O*
13. *S*
14.
15.

Part II

1. a. *S*
   b. $\underline{\text{c/o}}$:
   c. C/o intermittent $\textcircled{L}$ lateral knee pain.
2. a. *O*
   b. $\underline{\text{Sensation}}$:
   c. $\downarrow$ in $\textcircled{L}$ L5 dermatome.
3. a. *S*
   b. $\underline{\text{Hx}}$:
   c. States hx of arthroscope $\textcircled{R}$ knee of 02/02/94.
4. a. *S*
   b. $\underline{\text{Hx}}$:
   c. States hx of craniotomy in Feb. 1994.
5. a. *O*
   b. $\underline{\text{PROM}}$: **or** $\textcircled{R}$ LE:
   c. $\underline{\text{PROM}}$: WNL throughout $\textcircled{R}$ LE. **or** $\textcircled{R}$ LE: PROM WNL throughout.

Part III

The Physical Therapy Note:

Dx: Fx $\textcircled{L}$ femoral neck 01/12/94. $\textcircled{R}$ hip prosthesis inserted 01/14/94.
S: $\underline{\text{C/o}}$: C/o pain $\textcircled{R}$ while standing. $\underline{\text{Hx}}$: States fell at home & hit $\textcircled{R}$ hip on side of bathtub. Denies prior Rx by PT. $\underline{\text{Prior level of function}}$: Amb indep PTA; denies prior use of an assistive device. $\underline{\text{Home situation}}$: States lives alone in an apartment that is accessible by elevator; needs to amb curbs. $\underline{\text{Pt. goals}}$: Would like to return to home $\bar{p}$ D/C. Would like to eventually amb. indep $\bar{s}$ device.

O: <u>Amb</u>: // bars c̄ min +1 assist. ~20 ft. x 1 c̄ 50% PWB Ⓡ LE. Pt. became dizzy & nauseated p̄ 20 ft. of amb; nursing floor was notified & Pt. was returned to her room immediately. <u>Transfers</u>: Supine ↔ sit & w/c ↔ mat pivot transfer c̄ mod +1 assist. Sit ↔ stand c̄ min +1 assist. Ⓡ LE: AROMs limited 2° post-op restrictions; hip flex. 0–90°, hip abd. WNL, 0° hip internal & external rotation & adduction. All other AROMs WNL. STRENGTH: At least F throughout; not further assessed on this date due to recent surgery. <u>UEs & Ⓛ LE</u>: AROMs WNL except −5° Ⓡ elbow ext. STRENGTH: G+ throughout (group muscle test performed).

The Occupational Therapy Note:

Dx: Fx Ⓛ femoral neck 01/12/94. Ⓡ hip prosthesis inserted 01/14/94.

S: <u>C/o</u>: C/o pain Ⓡ hip while standing. <u>Hx</u>: States fell at home & hit Ⓡ hip on side of bathtub. <u>Prior level of function</u>: Amb indep PTA; denies prior use of an assistive device. <u>Home situation</u>: States lives alone in an apartment that is accessible by elevator; has no tub chair or portable commode at home. <u>Pt. goals</u>: Would like to return to home p̄ D/C. Would like to groom & dress indep but would "settle" for Meals on Wheels.

O: <u>Bathing</u>: UEs & trunk indep; min +1 assist. for LEs and needs set-up for sponge bath. <u>Grooming</u>: Seen B/S initially for assessment. Indep c̄ combing hair & caring for her teeth. Cares for her contact lenses indep from the w/c. <u>Transfers</u>: Supine ↔ sit & w/c ↔ bed c̄ mod +1 assist. <u>UEs</u>: APPEARANCE: IV infusing Ⓛ forearm. STRENGTH: G+ throughout bilat. (group muscle test). AROM: WNL except −5° Ⓡ elbow ext. FINE MOTOR SKILLS functional for ADL skills.

The Physical Therapy Functional Outcomes Note:

Dx: Fx Ⓛ femoral neck 01/12/94. Ⓡ hip prosthesis inserted 01/14/94.

S: <u>C/o</u>: C/o pain Ⓡ hip while standing. <u>Prior level of function</u>: Amb indep PTA; denies prior use of an assistive device. <u>Home situation</u>: States lives alone in an apartment that is accessible by elevator; needs to amb curbs. <u>Pt. goals</u>: Would like to return to home p̄ D/C. Would like to eventually amb indep s̄ device.

O: FUNCTIONAL LIMITATIONS: <u>Amb</u>: // bars c̄ min +1 assist. ~20 ft. x 1 c̄ 50% PWB ⓇLE. Pt. became dizzy & nauseated p̄ 20 ft. of amb; nursing floor was notified & Pt. was returned to her room immediately. <u>Transfers</u>: Supine ↔ sit & w/c ↔ mat pivot transfer c̄ mod +1 assist. Sit ↔ stand c̄ min +1 assist.
CAUSES OF FUNCTIONAL LIMITATIONS: Ⓡ LE: AROMs limited 2° post-op restrictions; hip flex. 0–90°, 0° hip internal & external rotation & adduction. STRENGTH: At least F throughout; not further assessed on this date due to recent surgery. UEs & Ⓛ LE: AROMs WNL except −5° Ⓡ elbow ext. STRENGTH: G+ throughout (group muscle test performed).

The Occupational Therapy Functional Outcomes Note:

Dx: Fx Ⓛ femoral neck 01/12/94. Ⓡ hip prosthesis inserted 01/14/94.

S: <u>C/o</u>: C/o pain Ⓡ hip while standing. <u>Prior level of function</u>: Amb indep PTA; denies prior use of an assistive device. <u>Home situation</u>: States lives alone in an apartment that is accessible by elevator; has no tub chair or portable commode at home. <u>Pt. goals</u>: Would like to return to home p̄ D/C. Would like to groom & dress indep but would "settle" for Meals on Wheels.

O: FUNCTIONAL LIMITATIONS: <u>Bathing</u>: UEs indep; min +1 assist. for LEs and needs set-up for sponge bath. <u>Grooming</u>: Seen B/S initially for assessment. Indep c̄ combing hair & caring for her teeth. Cares for her contact lenses indep from the w/c. <u>Transfers</u>: Supine ↔ sit & w/c ↔ bed c̄ mod +1 assist.
CAUSES OF FUNCTIONAL LIMITATIONS: <u>UEs</u>: APPEARANCE: IV infusing Ⓛ arm. STRENGTH: G+ throughout bilat. (group muscle test). AROM: WNL except −5° Ⓡ elbow ext.

CHAPTER 8: Writing Assessment (*A*): I—The Problem List

WORKSHEET 1

Part I

A: <u>Problem List</u>:
1. Dependence in transfers
2. Dependence in amb
3. Ⓡ hip pain while standing
4. ↓ Ⓡ elbow ext. AROM

Now formulate the problem list:
A. Ⓡ hip pain while standing
B. ↓ Ⓡ elbow ext. AROM
C.
D.
E. Dependence in transfers
F. Dependence in amb

Part II

Dx: CHF. <u>Hx</u>: ASHD, degenerative arthritis.
S: <u>C/o</u>: Generalized weakness & fatigue. No further assessment performed 2° Pt.'s mental status.
O: <u>Amb</u>: FWB in // bars for 1 min. x 2 c̄ min assist of 1. Fatigued p̄ standing x 2. All other assessment deferred 2° mental status. <u>Transfers</u>: Sit ↔ stand

c̄ min assist. of 1. <u>LE & UE AROM & PROM</u> WNL except for −90° shoulder abd. & −100° shoulder flex. bilat. <u>LE & UE strength</u> at least 3/5 (group muscle test); unable to further assess 2° Pt.'s mental status. <u>Mental status</u>: Oriented to person only, not to place, time, or date. At times combative & argumentative while in therapy. (Note: This version of the note varies from the version written on the worksheet itself. This was done to show you the variations that are acceptable for this note.)

A: <u>Problem List</u>:
1. Dependence in transfers
2. Dependence in amb
3. ↓ endurance
4. ↓ shoulder flex & abd ROM bilat.

Now formulate the problem list:
A.
B. dependence in transfers
C.
D. ↓ shoulder flex. & abd. ROM bilat.
E. dependence in amb
F. ↓ endurance
G.

CHAPTER 8: Writing Assessment (*A*): I—The Problem List

WORKSHEET 2

Part I

A. <u>Problem List</u>:
1. Dependence in transfers
2. Dependence in amb
3. Pain at incision site

Now formulate the problem list:
A. Pain at incision site
B.
C.
D. Dependence in transfers
E. Dependence in amb
F.

Dx: 17 y/o ♀ c̄ fx ℞ prox femur on (date). ORIF c̄ long plate & screws on (date).

S: C/o difficulty moving ℞ LE. <u>Hx</u>: Denies use of assist. device PTA. <u>Home situation</u>: Lives c̄ parents & 2 older siblings. <u>Prior level of function</u>: Very active in horseback riding & in organizations in school. <u>Pt. goals</u>: (Short term) to amb 17 steps c̄ crutches plus long distances to be able to return to school ASAP p̄ D/C. (Long term) to return to horseback riding.

O: FUNCTIONAL STATUS: <u>Transfers</u> supine ↔ sit indep; sit ↔ supine, sit ↔ stand in // bars, & w/c ↔ mat c̄ min +1 assist. <u>Amb</u> in // bars NWB ℞ LE for ~2 min. x 3 c̄ min +1 assist.

A: <u>Problem List</u>:
1. Dependence in transfers
2. Dependence in amb

CHAPTER 9: Writing Assessment (*A*): II—Long Term Goals

WORKSHEET 1

Part I

1. a. Pt. (unwritten and assumed)
   b. Use & manage w/c
   c. At home
   d. Indep (observable)
      Unlimited use (observable)
      Within 3 mo. (time span)

   Included in a functional outcomes reporting format? Yes, the need for this activity at home is stated within the goal itself.

2. a. Pt.
   b. Amb
   c. c̄ prosthesis
      s̄ device
      Level surfaces will be even & uneven
   d. Within 2 wks. (time span)
      At least 14 stairs (measurable)
      At least 1/2 mi. (measurable)
      Indep. (observable)

   Included in a functional outcomes reporting format? Yes, the need for this activity at home is added in a functional statement that is part of the goal: to assure Pt.'s ability to amb in & out of his home & around his yard.

3. a. Pt.
   b. Demonstrate AROM of the trunk
   c. A consistent method of measurement is assumed but is not written
   d. Full AROM (measurable)
      Pain-free AROM (measurable per Pt. reporting on a pain scale)
      4 wks. (time span)

   Included in a functional outcomes reporting format? Yes, because the tie to patient function is included in the goal: to prevent further injury while lifting, bending, & turning on his job.

4. a. Pt.
   b. Will demonstrate rolling
   c.
   d. The rolling must be segmental (observable)
      1 yr. (time span)

   Included in a functional outcomes reporting format? Maybe. If the patient were a small child, rolling might be considered a functional activity. However, 1 year is long time to work on rolling. This goal could be improved by stating what rolling would enable the patient to be able to do (repositioning self to prevent skin problems, allow less care by the caretaker, enable patient to start working on functional activities in supine or prone).

Part II

1. Pt. will indep amb NWB Ⓛ LE c̄ a walker on level surfaces for 40 ft. x 2 & 1-step elevation p̄ 2 wks. to allow Pt. to get around her house for ADLs.
2. Pt. will indep & correctly demonstrate care & wrapping of her residual limb c̄ elastic wrap 100% of the time within 2 wks. to prepare for prosthetic training.
3. Pt. will ↑ Ⓡ shouder flex & abd AROM to 120° within 2 mo. to improve Pt.'s ability to reach items on the shelves in her kitchen & closets at home during ADL.
4. Pt. will demonstrate correct use of pursed lip breathing pattern during amb & performance of daily exercise program 100% of the time to ↑ her efficiency & ability to perform all ADL. (Note: A time span for this goal is missing & should be added to the goal.)

Part III

1. ↑ ability of Pt.'s Ⓡ UE to lift the pots & pans in her kitchen to that of her Ⓛ UE within 1 mo. of Rx.

Included in a functional outcomes reporting format? Yes, particularly if Pt. was seen in the home setting where the ability level could be observed.

2. ↑ Pt.'s ability to reach items in the overhead cabinet of her kitchen with her Ⓡ UE to that of the Ⓛ UE within 1 mo.

Included in a functional outcomes reporting format? Yes, this goal is very functional.

3. ↑ Ⓡ elbow flexion AROM to −3 to −5° of WNL within 2 mo.

Included in a functional outcomes reporting format? No, this goal is not functional in nature.

4. ↑ Ⓡ biceps strength to G to N within 2 mo.

Included in a functional outcomes reporting format? No, this goal is not functional in nature.

CHAPTER 9: Writing Assessment (A): II—Long Term Goals

WORKSHEET 2

Part I

1. a. Pt. (assumed since it is not stated)
   b. Amb

c. c̄ straight cane
   On level surfaces
   On stairs
d. Indep (observable)
   150 ft. x 2 (measurable)
   At least 5 stairs (measurable)
   Within 2 wks. (time span)

Included in a functional outcomes reporting format? Yes, this goal includes a statement that ties this goal to function at home: so Pt.'s level of indep at home ↑ s.

2. a. Pt. (assumed)
   b. ↑ Ⓛ ankle AROM
   c. It is assumed a goniometer will be used to measure the Pt.'s ankle AROM.
   d. To WNL (measurable)
      Within 1 mo. (time span)

Included in a functional outcomes reporting format? Maybe. Normally, impairments in AROM would not be included. However, some facilities include impairments if the link between AROM and function is shown in the goal. While this goal states that ↑ AROM is needed to return Pt. to prior level of function at work, one must wonder if completely normal AROM is needed. If WNL AROM is needed, this goal could be included in some facilities. If completely normal AROM is not needed, this goal would not be included in a functional outcomes format at most facilities.

3. a. Pt.'s wife
   b. Transfer Pt.
   c. W/c ↔ supine in bed & w/c ↔ toilet are the type of transfers after 5 sessions of family teaching
   d. Min +1 assist. (observable)
      p̄ 2 mo. of Rx (time span)

Included in a functional outcomes reporting format? Yes. This activity is very functional and must be done if this patient is to remain at home in his wife's care.

Part II

1. Pt. will demonstrate good undisturbed sitting balance on the edge of a mat for at least 5 min. p̄ 2 mo. of Rx to allow Pt. to transfer better.
2. Pt. will indep transfer supine ↔ sit, sit ↔ stand, on/off toilet c̄ raised toilet seat p̄ 2 wks. of Rx.
3. In order to speed Pt.'s rate of recovery, Pt. will correctly explain rationale for & importance of performing AROM exercises daily p̄ 1 wk. of Rx.
4. Pt. will indep propel w/c on tiled & carpeted level surfaces p̄ 2 mo. of Rx.

Part III

Long Term Goals
1. Pt. will return to previous WNL gait pattern within 2 mo.

2. ↑ Ⓛ hip AROM to WNL in 1 mo. to enable Pt. to return to her gymnastics class.
3. ↑ Ⓛ hip musculature strength to 4–5/5 within 2 mo. to enable Pt. to safely return to her gymnastics class.

Functional Limitations:
1. Abnormal gait pattern.
2. Inability to function in her gymnastics class because of limited Ⓛ hip AROM & Ⓛ hip musculature strength.

Anticipated Functional Outcomes:
1. Pt. will return to previous WNL gait pattern within 2 mo.
2. Pt. will be able to function in her gymnastics class.

CHAPTER 10: Writing Assessment (A): III—Short Term Goals

WORKSHEET 1

Part I

1. a. Pt.
   b. ↑ Ⓡ shoulder flexion AROM
   c. It is assumed a goniometer would be used to measure AROM
   d. 0–90° (measurable)
   Within 6 Rx sessions (time span)
   To enable Pt. to reach her overhead kitchen cabinet shelves (functional)

Included in a functional outcomes reporting format? Maybe. It might not be if the facility refused to include impairments such as ROM. It might be if the facility included impairments as they related to function.

2. a. Pt.
   b. Will grasp object in midline
   c. Object will be in midline
   d. 3 out of 4 times (observable)
   Within 3 mo. (time span)
   In order to ↑ the Pt.'s functional use of his UEs during ADLs (functional)

Included in a functional outcomes reporting format? Yes. This goal could be made better by stating which ADL activities specifically would improve with improvement of this ability to grasp in midline.

3. a. Pt.
   b. Will demonstrate good body mechanics
   c.
   d. Correct performance of at least 90% of tasks in obstacle course (observable, measurable) p̄ 3 Rx sessions (time span)

In order to prevent further Pt. injury (functional)

Included in a functional outcomes reporting format? Yes. This goal could be improved by describing the obstacle course as an obstacle course of functional activities needed for the Pt.'s ADLs (if that is true).

Part II

1. Pt. will indep amb c̄ a walker on level surfaces only NWB Ⓛ LE ~100 ft. p̄ 1 wk. of Rx.
2. Pt.'s wife & son will indep transfer Pt. w/c ↔ supine in bed p̄ 4 family training sessions.
3. Pt. will indep wrap residual limb c̄ Ace wrap p̄ 5 Rx sessions to prepare his residual limb for prosthetic training.

Part III

1. Pt. will don/doff prosthesis with standby assist. of 1 person within 1 wk.

Included in a functional outcomes reporting format? Yes. This is a functional activity that has been tied to ambulation.

2. Within 1 wk. Pt. will stand in // bars c̄ min +1 assist & verbal cues c̄ at least half of his body wt. shifting onto Ⓛ LE.

Included in a functional outcomes reporting format? Yes. Ambulation is a functional skill.

3. Within 2 days Pt. will tolerate prone-on-elbows position for 5 min.

Included in a functional outcomes reporting format? No. This is a necessary activity, but this goal is not currently tied to a functional activity.

Part IV

1. Degree (time span, measurable factors)
2. Degree (time span, measurable or observable factor—could be assumed to be 100% of the time correctly)
3. Audience, Behavior (who will do what?)

CHAPTER 10: Writing Assessment (A): III—Short Term Goals

WORKSHEET 2

Part I

1. a. Pt.
   b. Will ↑ cardiopulmonary endurance
   c. p̄ amb. for 150 ft.
   d. Max ↑ resp. rate of 5 resp/min. (measurable) p̄ 6 Rx sessions (time span)

Included in a functional outcomes reporting format? No. This statement is not closely enough tied to function and does not show that the patient needs the care of a therapist to achieve the goal.

2. a. Pt.
    b. Will be able to long sit
    c. Propped c̄ a pillow or wedge
    d. Maintaining good head position 0–45° neck flex. for 1 min. (observable)
       Within 6 wks. of Rx (time span)

Included in a functional outcomes reporting format? Yes. However, this goal could be much improved if the therapist could state some ADLs the Pt. would be able to perform if the Pt. achieved this goal.

3. a. Pt.
    b. Will transfer supine ↔ sit
    c. On a mat
    d. Using rotation & pushing c̄ his UEs (observable)
       1 out of 3 attempts correct (observable)
       Within 2 mo. (time span)

Included in a functional outcomes reporting format? Yes. This could be made better if tied to a longer term functional goal.

Part II

1. While Pt. is in supine position, Pt. will hold head erect in midline for 15 sec. within 3 mo. of Rx.
2. Pt. will roll supine ↔ prone on a mat indep in 6–8 wks.
3. Pt. will amb 5 stairs c̄ a walker 50% PWB Ⓡ LE c̄ min assist from his wife within 1 wk.

Part III

1. Pt. will tolerate 7 reps of both UE PNF diagonals c̄ a rise in pulse of 20 beats/min. or less within 1 wk. of Rx to ↑ Pt.'s ability to use UEs in ADL.
   Another acceptable manner: Pt. will perform 7 reps. of bilat. UE PNF diagonals.
   Functional Limitations: ↓ ability to retrieve items from overhead cupboards.
   Expected Functional Outcomes: Pt. will be able to retrieve items from overhead cupboards.
   Short Term Goal: Pt. will be able to perform 7 reps of both PNF diagonals to ↑ her ability to use her UEs in retrieving items from overhead cupboards.
2. ↑ cervical rotation AROM to 0–10° bilat. in 2 days.
3. Pt. will amb c̄ crutches NWB Ⓡ LE for 40 ft. x 2 on level surfaces c̄ min +1 assist. within 1 wk.
   Another acceptable manner: Pt. will amb on level surfaces NWB Ⓡ LE c̄ crutches for 40 ft. x 2 c̄ +1 min assist.

Part IV

1. Degree (time span), Audience (could be assumed)

2. Degree (how much AROM is expected? Also, tying it into function would be helpful), Audience (could be assumed)
3. Audience, Behavior (ambulate?), Degree (time span, numbers of stairs)

CHAPTER 11: Writing Assessment (A): IV—Summary

WORKSHEET 1

Part I

1. *O*
2. *S*
3. *S*
4. *S*
5. *A*
6.
7. *A*
8. *A*
9.
10. *A*
11. *S*
12. *O*
13. *O*
14.
15. *O*
16. *S*
17. Prob.
18.
19. *O*
20. *A*
21.
22. *S*

Part II

1. Summary
2. Prob. List
3. Short
4. Short
5. Prob. List
6. Summary
7. Prob. List
8. Long
9. Long
10. Summary
11. Long
12. Prob. List
13. Long
14. Short
15. Short
16. Prob. List
17. Summary

Part III

1. Pt. has poor potential to be w/c indep.
2. Pt. did not follow commands because Pt. is HOH.
3. Pt. did not answer questions directly during initial interview.

CHAPTER 11: Writing Assessment (A): IV—Summary

WORKSHEET 2

Part I

1. *S*
2. *A*
3. *O*
4. *O*
5. *O*
6.
7. *O*
8. *S*
9. *A*
10. *A*
11.
12. *S*
13. *A*
14. *S*
15.
16.
17. *O*

Part II

1. Long
2. Summary
3. Short
4. Short
5. Prob. List
6. Short
7. Short
8. Prob. List
9. Long
10. Summary
11. Prob. List
12. Long
13. Summary
14. Long
15. Summary
16. Prob. List

Part III

1. Interview was difficult to complete 2° Pt.'s distractibility & incessant talking.
2. Initial assessment not completed 2° Pt.'s bowel movement while amb.
3. Pt. has potential to be indep in w/c propulsion & management but does not have potential for amb.

Review Worksheet: SOA

Part I

1. ® hip pain, worse when moving
2. No knowledge of precautions for THR pts.
3. Dependent transfers
4.
5. ↓ Ⓛ LE strength
6a. ↓ ® LE strength
6b. ↓ ® LE AROM
7. Dependent amb

Part II

Dx: Degenerative joint disease ® hip; THR on (date).

S: <u>C/o</u>: ® hip pain in area of sutures; reports intensity of 3 when sitting & 7 when moving (0 = no pain, 10 = worst pain). <u>Prior level of function</u>: Amb s̄ assist. device immediately PTA. Pt. is retired; hobby is gardening. States no knowledge of precautions for Pts. c̄ THR. <u>Pt. goals</u>: Short term: To return home c̄ wife p̄ D/C. Long term: To return to gardening & yard work activities. <u>Hx</u>: Ⓛ THR 01/10/94. Pain level ® hip was 9–10 on pain scale & constant PTA. <u>Home situation</u>: Lives c̄ wife in his own home. Describes 1 step to enter c̄ railing on ® ascending. Owns a 3-in-1 commode, walker, & cane.

O: <u>Transfers</u>: Supine ↔ sit c̄ min +1 assist. Sit ↔ stand & w/c ↔ mat pivot c̄ mod +1 assist. Toilet transfers not assessed on this date. <u>Amb</u>: Stood 10% PWB Ⓡ LE in // bars c̄ mod +1 assist. for 1 min. x 2. <u>UEs & Ⓛ LE</u>: AROM WNL throughout. STRENGTH: G+ throughout UEs bilat; G throughout Ⓛ LE (group muscle test performed). Ⓡ LE: INCISION of 10 cm length over greater trochanter noted; healing well. AROM of ankle WNL. PROM: −20° hip flex, 0–10° hip abd, 0° hip ext; hip add. internal & external rotation not tested 2° hip precautions & recent surgery. Knee ext/flex: 0–70°. STRENGTH: Grossly T in hip & knee musculature; ankle dorsiflexion G+/N, ankle plantarflexion at least P but not tested further 2° Pt.'s NWB Ⓡ LE status.

A: Pt. has good rehab. potential, although progress will be somewhat slowed 2° Pt.'s pneumonia.

<u>Problem List:</u>
1. Lack of knowledge of precautions for Pts. c̄ THR
2. Dependent transfers
3. Dependent amb
4. ↓ Ⓛ LE strength
5. ↓ Ⓡ LE strength
6. ↓ Ⓡ LE AROM
7. Ⓛ hip pain

<u>Long Term Goals:</u>
1. Pt. will indep state & demonstrate precautions for Pts. c̄ THR within 2 wks. of Rx.
2. Indep transfers sit ↔ stand, supine ↔ sit, w/c ↔ mat & on/off toilet within 2 wks.
3. Indep amb c̄ walker on level surfaces & 1-step elevation within 2 wks.
4. G+ to N (4+ to 5/5) strength Ⓛ LE within 2 wks.
5. At least F (3/5) strength Ⓡ hip flexors, extensors, abductors & adductors within 2 wks.
6. Pain-free AROM Ⓡ hip flex. 0–90° & WNL hip abd. & ext. within 2 wks.

<u>Short Term Goals:</u>
1. Pt. will be able to state correctly the precautions for Pts. c̄ THR whenever asked within 3 days.
2. ↓ dependence in transfers sit ↔ stand & w/c ↔ mat pivot to min +1 p̄ 3 days of Rx.
3. Indep transfers supine ↔ sit in 1 wk.
4. Pt. will amb in // bars c̄ min +1 assist. for 20 ft. x 2 within 3 days.
5. Pt. will indep demonstrate Ⓛ LE exercise program to be performed in his room within 3 days of Rx to promote quick return to indep amb.
6. ↑ strength Ⓛ LE to G+ (4+/5) in 1 wk.
7. At least P strength Ⓡ hip & knee musculature within 1 wk.
8. Ⓡ hip flex. 0–90° & WNL hip abd. & ext. c̄ Pt.'s report of pain at a level of 5 or less on pain scale (0 = no pain, 10 = worst possible pain) within 1 wk.

Part III

Dx: Degenerative joint disease Ⓡ hip; THR on (date).

S: <u>C/o</u>: Ⓡ hip pain in area of sutures; reports intensity of 3 when sitting & 7 when moving (0 = no pain, 10 = worst pain). <u>Prior level of function</u>: Amb s̄ assist. device immediately PTA. Pt. is retired; hobby is gardening. States no knowledge of precautions for pts. c̄ THR. <u>Pt. goals</u>: Short term: To return home c̄ wife p̄ D/C. Long term: To return to gardening & yard work activities. <u>Home situation</u>: Lives c̄ wife in his own home. Describes 1 step to enter c̄ railing on Ⓡ ascending. Owns a 3-in-1 commode, walker, & cane.

O: FUNCTIONAL STATUS: <u>Transfers</u>: Supine ↔ sit c̄ min +1 assist. Sit ↔ stand & w/c ↔ mat pivot c̄ mod +1 assist. <u>Amb</u>: Stood 10% PWB Ⓡ LE in // bars c̄ mod +1 assist. for 1 min. x 2. CAUSES OF FUNCTIONAL LIMITATIONS: <u>UEs & Ⓛ LE</u>: STRENGTH: G throughout Ⓛ LE (group muscle test performed). Ⓡ LE: INCISION of 10 cm length over greater trochanter noted; healing well. PROM: −20° hip flex, 0–10° hip abd, 0° hip ext; hip add. Knee ext/flex: 0–70°. STRENGTH grossly T in hip & knee musculature.

A: Pt. has good rehab. potential, although progress will be somewhat slowed 2° Pt.'s pneumonia.

Functional Limitations:

1. Lack of knowledge of precautions for Pts. c̄ THR.
2. Dependent transfers.
3. Dependent amb.

Expected Functional Outcomes:

1. Pt. will indep state & demonstrate precautions for pts. c̄ THR within 2 wks. of Rx.
2. Indep transfers sit ↔ stand, supine ↔ sit, w/c ↔ mat & on/off toilet within 2 wks.
3. Indep amb c̄ walker on level surfaces & 1-step elevation within 2 wks.

Short Term Goals:

1. Pt. will be able to state correctly the precautions for Pts. c̄ THR whenever asked within 3 days.
2. ↓ dependence in transfers sit ↔ stand & w/c ↔ mat pivot to min +1 p̄ 3 days of Rx.
3. Indep transfers supine ↔ sit in 1 wk.
4. Pt. will amb in // bars c̄ min +1 assist. for 20 ft. x 2 within 3 days.
5. Pt. will indep demonstrate Ⓛ LE exercise program to be performed in his room within 3 days of Rx to promote quick return to indep amb.

CHAPTER 12: Writing Plan (*P*)

WORKSHEET 1

Part I

1. *A*
2. *P*
3. *S*
4. *O*
5. *S*
6. *A*
7. *P*
8. *S*
9. *S*
10. *O*
11. Prob.
12. *P*
13. *A*
14. *S*
15. *P*
16. *S*
17. *A*
18. *O*
19. *P*
20. *O*
21. *A*
22. *A* or *O* (your opinion or fact?)

Part II

1. Pt. will receive hot pack to lumbar area for 20 min. BID.
2. Pt. will receive US to Ⓡ upper trapezius at 1.0 W/cm² for 7 min. OD.
3. BID: Pt. will be progressed through attached home exercise program.

Part III

1. How often
   For how long
   Setting of the pump
   To what (UE? LE?)
2. For how long
   Which whirlpool
   Temperature
   To which part of the body
   Some facilities list type of agitation (full, mild, etc.)

CHAPTER 12: Writing Plan (*P*)

WORKSHEET 2

Part I

1. *O*
2. *P*
3. *A*
4. *S*
5. *A*
6. *O*
7. *S*
8. *S*
9. *A*
10. *P*
11. *S*
12. *O*
13. *S*
14. *P*
15. *A*

16. *O*
17. *P*
18. *A*

Part II

1. **P:** Will be seen 3x/wk. as an O.P. for the following: Pulsed US to ℞ shoulder at 1.5 W/cm² for 7 min.; mobilization to ℞ shoulder; ice pack for 20 min. Will instruct Pt. in a home exercise program (attached). Will request OT consult.

2. **P:** Will be seen by PT BID for the following: PROM exercises to LEs beginning c̄ 10 reps each & ↑ reps to tolerance; gait training c̄ axillary crutches NWB ℞ LE; transfer training. Will be instructed in proper care & wrapping of his residual limb.

Review Worksheet: SOAP

Part II

Formulate a problem list:
2. a. Pain ℞ ankle
     Pain ℞ shoulder
   b.
   c. ↓ ℞ elbow AAROM
   d. Pt. at risk for ↓ AROM ℞ hand & wrist
   e. Dependent transfers
   f. Dependent w/c management
   g. Dependent w/c propulsion

Review Worksheet: SOAP Answer Sheet

Dx: Fx ℞ distal tibia & ℞ prox. humerus. Cast applied to tibia; ℞ humerus immobilized by a sling.

S: <u>C/o:</u> Pain ℞ ankle while in a dependent position & severe pain ℞ shoulder c̄ elbow AAROM. <u>Prior level of function:</u> States never used a w/c before. Active; indep in amb s̄ device or previously noted deviation. Pt. is ℞-handed dominant. <u>Home situation:</u> Lives c̄ parents in a 1-story house c̄ 1 step at entrance; home has carpeting throughout. <u>School situation:</u> All on 1 level c̄ no steps to enter the school; floor surfaces are linoleum. Distances between classrooms are up to 1500 ft. long. Has 7 class periods/day. <u>Pt. goals:</u> Is a high school student & wants to return to school ASAP p̄ D/C. States school is very challenging & competitive & does not believe she can afford to stay out of school until fx are healed.

O: <u>Transfers:</u> Sit ↔ stand & w/c ↔ mat c̄ max +1 assist. Supine ↔ sit c̄ mod +1 assist. Toilet transfers not yet assessed. <u>Amb:</u> Not feasible at this time. <u>W/c management:</u> Unable to manage ℞ w/c brakes or leg rests. <u>W/c propulsion:</u> Propelled w/c using Ⓛ LE & UE 10 ft. ā fatiguing c̄ min +1 assist. & verbal cues. <u>Ⓛ UE & LE:</u> WNL AROM & strength. <u>℞ UE:</u> Pt. is NWB ℞ UE. ℞ shoulder not assessed due to fx. ℞ elbow AAROM is 30–70°; strength grossly P in biceps & triceps. ℞ hand & wrist AROM very slow but WNL; strength grossly P in musculature controlling ℞ hand & wrist. <u>℞ LE:</u> AROM WNL & strength N at hip & knee. Short leg cast ℞ ankle & foot so not assessed; Pt. is NWB ℞ LE. Toes warm & normal color; able to wiggle toes. Cried 2° pain when ℞ ankle placed initially in a dependent position.

A: Further assessment of toilet transfers is needed. Pt. should progress quickly, but Pt. will need assist. c̄ w/c propulsion at school until her endurance improves. Pt. needs much encouragement to complete AROM ℞ wrist & hand.

<u>Problem List:</u>
1. Dependent transfers
2. Dependent w/c management
3. Dependent w/c propulsion
4. ↓ ℞ elbow AAROM
5. Pt. at risk for ↓ AROM ℞ hand & wrist

6. Pain ® shoulder
7. Pain ® ankle

Long Term Goals:
1. Indep pain-free transfers w/c ↔ mat, supine ↔ sit, sit ↔ stand, & on/off toilet in 10 days.
2. Indep management of w/c brakes & leg rests in 10 days.
3. Indep w/c propulsion on linoleum & carpeted surfaces for ~100 ft. in 10 days.
4. Indep in ® elbow self-ROM exercises in 10 days.
5. ® elbow AROM of 15–90° in 10 days.
6. Full pain-free AROM of ® wrist & fingers in 10 days.

Short Term Goals: To be achieved in 5 days
1. Pt. will transfer sit ↔ stand & w/c ↔ mat c̄ min +1 assist.
2. Pt. will transfer supine ↔ sit c̄ standby assist. of 1.
3. Pt. will manage w/c brakes & leg rests c̄ mod assist. of 1 & verbal cues.
4. Pt. will propel w/c ~50 ft. c̄ verbal cues only.
5. Pt. will require verbal cues to perform ® elbow self-ROM exercises.
6. ↑ ® elbow AROM to 25–80°.
7. Pt. will be able to perform AROM exercises to ® wrist & fingers indep.

P: BID: Transfers on/off toilet will be assessed. Transfer training w/c ↔ mat, supine ↔ sit, sit ↔ stand, & on/off toilet. Training in w/c management & propulsion. AAROM exercises ® elbow, AROM exercises ® wrist & fingers. Pt. will be instructed in self-ROM exercises ® elbow & AROM exercises ® wrist & fingers to be performed at home.

Review Worksheet: SOAP Answer Sheet— Functional Outcomes Format

Dx: Fx ® distal tibia & ® prox. humerus. Cast applied to tibia; ® humerus immobilized by a sling.

S: Prior level of function: States never used a w/c before. Active; indep in amb s̄ device or previously noted deviation. Pt. is ®-handed dominant. Home situation: Lives c̄ parents in a 1-story house c̄ 1 step at entrance; home has carpeting throughout. School situation: All on 1 level c̄ no steps to enter the school; floor surfaces are linoleum. Distances between classrooms are up to 1500 ft. long. Has 7 class periods/day. Pt. goals: Is a high school student & wants to return to school ASAP p̄ D/C. States school is very challenging & competitive & does not believe she can afford to stay out of school until fx are healed.

O: FUNCTIONAL STATUS: Transfers: Sit ↔ stand & w/c ↔ mat c̄ max +1 assist. Supine ↔ sit c̄ mod +1 assist. Toilet transfers not yet assessed. Amb: Not feasible at this time. W/c management: Unable to manage ® w/c brakes or leg rests. W/c propulsion: Propelled w/c using Ⓛ LE & UE 10 ft. ā fatiguing c̄ min +1 assist. & verbal cues. CAUSES OF FUNCTIONAL PROBLEMS: ® UE: Pt. is NWB ® UE. ® shoulder not asessed due to fx. ® elbow AAROM is 30–70°; strength grossly P in biceps & triceps. ® hand & wrist AROM very slow but WNL; strength grossly P in musculature controlling ® hand & wrist. ® LE: Short leg cast ® ankle & foot so not assessed; Pt. is NWB ® LE. Cried 2° pain when ® ankle placed initially in a dependent position.

A: Further assessment of toilet transfers is needed. Pt. should progress quickly, but Pt. will need assist. c̄ w/c propulsion at school until her endurance improves. Pt. needs much encouragement to complete AROM ® wrist & hand.

Functional Limitations:
1. Dependent transfers
2. Dependent w/c management
3. Dependent w/c propulsion
4. Non-functional ® hand & wrist

Expected Functional Outcomes:
1. Indep pain-free transfers w/c ↔ mat, supine ↔ sit, sit ↔ stand, & on/off toilet in 10 days.
2. Indep management of w/c brakes & leg rests in 10 days.
3. Indep w/c propulsion on linoleum & carpeted surfaces for ~100 ft. in 10 days.
4. Functional Ⓡ hand & wrist

Short Term Goals: To be achieved in 5 days
1. Pt. will transfer sit ↔ stand & w/c ↔ mat c̄ min +1 assist.
2. Pt. will transfer supine ↔ sit c̄ standby assist. of 1.
3. Pt. will manage w/c brakes & leg rests c̄ mod assist of 1 & verbal cues.
4. Pt. will propel w/c ~50 ft. c̄ verbal cues only.
5. Pt. will be able to perform AROM exercises to Ⓡ wrist & finger indep.

P: BID: Transfers on/off toilet will be assessed. Transfer training w/c ↔ mat, supine ↔ sit, sit ↔ stand, & on/off toilet. Training in w/c management & propulsion. Pt. will be instructed in self-ROM exercises Ⓡ elbow & AROM exercises Ⓡ wrist & fingers to be performed at home.

Note Writing and the Problem-Solving Process

PROBLEM-SOLVING PROCESS*	WHAT THE THERAPIST DOES	PORTION OF THE NOTE
1. Identify the problem	A. Reads the chart	INITIAL NOTE Problem or Diagnosis
	B. Interviews the patient	Subjective (*S*)
	C. Plans the objective measurements to be performed	(Not documented)
	D. Carries out the objective measurements and observations planned	Objective (*O*)
	E. Interprets the information in the Problem, *S*, and *O* portions of the note to identify factors that are *not* WNL; a PT diagnosis may be made	Assessment (*A*) Problem List
	F. Together with the patient, establishes goals for	
	(1) How the patient's problems will be resolved following the entire program of therapy intervention	Long Term Goals
	(2) What can be achieved within a short period of time; the first steps toward achieving the long term goals	Short Term Goals
2. Identify and locate resources	G. Identifies limitations and/or assets that may help or hinder the patient's progress	Impressions or Summary
3. Identify alternative courses a. Plus and minus aspects of each b. Possible outcomes of each	H. Considers all of the possible treatments to achieve each short term goal (and the long term goals); looks at the positive and negative aspects of each; weighs factors such as efficiency of time and money	(At times documented under Impressions in the assessment (*A*) portion of the note)

167

168

4. Select course of action	I. Formulates a treatment plan	Plan (P)
5. Initiates course of action	J. Begins treatment	(Documented in daily notes required by some third-party payers, usually under O)
6. Collect data	K. Reassesses patient by further patient interview and objective measurements during and after treatment (ongoing process)	INTERIM NOTE Subjective (S) Objective (O)
7. Evaluate	L. Looks at new information gathered and compares with former measurements, problem list, long and short term goals, and determines whether present treatment plan is appropriate or needs revision	Assessment (A) Summary (occasionally address long term goals and problem list)
	M. Revises short term goals	Short term goals
8. Repeats steps 3 and 4	N. Repeats steps H and I	Plan (P)
9. Continue with steps 5, 6, 7, 8, 9, and so forth	O. Continues with steps J, K, L, M, N, O, and so forth	NEW INTERIM NOTE Subjective (S) Objective (O) Assessment (A) Plan (P) as needed

*From Wolf, S: *Clinical Decision Making in Physical Therapy.* FA Davis, Philadelphia, 1985, with permission.

Summary of SOAP
Note Contents

The Problem

The Problem includes any of the following information that is relevant to the patient's present condition or treatment:

Diagnosis
Past surgeries
Past conditions or diseases
Present conditions or diseases
Test results
Recent or past surgery

Subjective

Subjective includes any of the following information given to the therapist by the patient or a designated family member:

The patient's history
The patient's level of function prior to onset of the current condition (prior level of function)
The patient's lifestyle or home situation
The patient's emotions or attitudes
The patient's goals
The patient's complaint(s)
The patient's response to treatment
Any other information that is relevant to the patient's case or present condition

INTERIM NOTES

Interim Notes include updates or additional information regarding the patient's status since the most recent note was written.

DISCHARGE SUMMARY

The *Discharge Summary* includes updates or additional information regarding the patient's status since the most recent note was written *or* completely summarizes the patient's complaints, home situation, whether the patient feels the goals set were achieved, and whether the patient feels ready to function at home.

Objective

Objective includes any of the following information (depending on the individual clinical facility):

1. Part of the patient's history taken from the medical record and relevant to the current problem (Note: Only certain facilities include information from the medical record under *O*).
2. Information that is a result of objective measurements or observations (must be measurable and reproducible data; may use data base, flow sheets, or charts and summarize data under *O*).
3. Part of the treatment already given to a patient (particularly specific exercises taught to the patient, the level of independence in performing the exercises, number of repetitions tolerated, positions used, modifications necessary).
4. Functional information; this information is usually stated first in the *O* section of the note.

INTERIM NOTES

Interim Notes update or add to the information reported in the initial note or last interim note.

DISCHARGE SUMMARY

The *Discharge Summary* updates the patient's status since the last note was written *or* completely summarizes the patient's condition upon discharge from the facility (more similar to the initial note in format and length).

Assessment

The **Assessment** includes four sections that, together, provide the reader with the therapist's reasoning for goals and treatment.

THE PROBLEM LIST

The *Problem List* provides a summary of the patient's major problems as written in the subjective and objective parts of the note. The steps to formulating the problem list are as follows:

1. (Prerequisite step:) Write the *S* and *O* portions of the note.
2. Review the *S* and *O* portions of the note, jotting down or highlighting finds that are WNL and that can be influenced or changed by therapy intervention. (Medical or psychiatric problems do *not* belong to the therapy problem list.)
3. Set priorities as to which problem is the most important, the next important, and so forth.
4. List the therapy problems in order of priority.

Interim Notes

Interim Notes list a problem only if it is a new problem *or* if it has been resolved.

Discharge Summary

The Discharge Summary notes whether a problem has been resolved or still exists.

LONG TERM GOALS

Long Term Goals

1. State the long term expected outcomes of therapy.
2. Are based on the therapy problem list (and/or on the PT diagnosis).
3. Are the basis for setting short term goals.

Components of long term goals:

Audience: The patient, a family member, or the patient with a family member (sometimes implied).

Behavior: An action verb, often followed by the object of the behavior.

Condition: The circumstances under which the behavior must be done or the conditions necessary for the behavior to occur (sometimes implied).

Degree: The minimal number, the percentage or proportion, limitation or departure from a fixed standard, or distinguishing features of successful performance; always includes a time span for achievement of the goal and a tie into the patient's functional status.

Interim Notes

Long term goals usually are not addressed in interim notes unless they have been achieved or need to be revised.

Discharge Summary

The discharge summary indicates which goals have been achieved and which have not been achieved (and why they were not achieved).

SHORT TERM GOALS

Short Term Goals

1. Are the steps along the way to achieving long term goals.
2. Are based on the long term goals.
3. Serve as the basis for treatment planning.

The components of short term goals are the same as those of long term goals. Short term goals differ from long term goals in that

1. The time span is not as long.
2. Short term goals are not as frequently expressed in functional terms in some facilities.
3. Short term goals are frequently revised.

Interim Notes

Interim notes refer to the short term goals achieved and set new short term goals. If a goal has not yet been achieved, the notes comment on the reason the short term goal has not been achieved and reset the goal to make it more reasonable or restate the same goal to include a new time span.

Discharge Summary

In some facilities, comments are made on the most recently set short term goals and why they were or were not achieved. In other facilities, no comment is made on the short term goals.

IMPRESSIONS OR SUMMARY

Impressions or Summary can include any of the following types of information:

The physical therapy diagnosis
Correlations between the subjective and objective information in the note

Justification for the goals and/or treatment plan
Clarification of the patient's major problems
Justification for further treatment
A discussion of the patient's progress (or lack of progress) in therapy
A discussion of the patient's rehab potential and why
An explanation of any difficulties in obtaining information during the initial interview and testing
Suggestions for further testing, treatment, or referrals needed

Plan

The *Plan* must include the following information:

1. Frequency per day or per week that the patient will be seen (or the total number of visits that the therapist will see the patient).
2. The treatment the patient will receive.

Also frequently included are the following:

3. The location of the treatment
4. The treatment progression
5. Plans for further assessment or reassessment
6. Plans for discharge
7. Patient and family education
8. Equipment needs and equipment ordered for or sold to the patient
9. Referral to other services; whether there are plans to consult with the patient's physician regarding further treatment or referral

INTERIM NOTES

The treatment plan will need to be revised as the patient's condition is reassessed and new short term goals are set.

DISCHARGE SUMMARY

The following information should be briefly stated:

1. What the treatment was
2. If instruction in a home program was done and the patient's level of independence in the program
3. If any other type of instruction of the patient or family was performed
4. If the patient was sold any type of equipment
5. If written instructions for any equipment sold to the patient were given
6. If a referral to a home health agency or any other professional was made
7. The number of times the patient was seen in therapy
8. Any instances of the patient skipping or canceling treatment sessions
9. If and when the patient was not seen or was put on hold and why
10. To where the patient is discharged
11. The reason for discharge
12. Recommendations for follow-up treatment or care given to the patient.

Tips for Note Writing for Third-Party Payers

Diagnosis

1. The current diagnosis and any relevant secondary diagnoses and/or test results should be included. At times, the relevant secondary diagnosis can help justify the need for assessment of a patient's functional level, even if the patient does not need prolonged OT or PT treatment.
2. The onset of the current diagnosis and the date that therapy began are essential to the D/C note.

Subjective

1. *Do not* list irrelevant information. Subjective information should help demonstrate the need for therapy.
2. When you report any complaints, keep the complaints brief and to the point. What does the patient see as his or her biggest problem? How does this problem tie into patient function (if the problem itself is not functional)?
3. Have the patient rate his or her subjective complaints on a scale. Use of a pain scale is one example. Functional abilities at home and the amount of assistance the patient required to do them (e.g., the number of people needed) is another. Subjective information put on a type of numeric scale can be used to re-evaluate the patient's progress.
4. Avoid listing nonspecific complaints in interim (progress) notes that are the result of normal patient depression or discouragement. Statements like "I don't think I'm doing very well" may serve as a red flag to the reviewers and may not be validated by the objective data.
5. *Do* list the patient level of functioning prior to the onset of his or her current diagnosis. This can help justify the need for treatment in the case of a chronic illness. It can also justify the need for teaching by the therapist. (For example, a patient who has never used a walker before will need instruction in its proper use.)
6. *Do* briefly describe the patient's home situation. Does the patient live alone? Who will be home during the day to care for the patient, if needed? Are there steps present, and is there

a railing? Are the steps essential for the patient to ambulate? What is the distance from the bed to the bathroom, to the kitchen, and so forth? Are the surfaces on the floors carpeted, tiled, linoleum, or hardwood, and are there any throw rugs present? Are there grab bars in the bathroom around the toilet or tub? Can a wheelchair fit through the doorways and/or turn in the rooms?

7. Briefly list any relevant history from the patient. Has the patient's functional status declined recently and why? Include whether the patient has received therapy before, why, and when. Also, has the patient ever used an assistive device before? Why and when? Does the patient own an assistive device or adaptive equipment?

8. Find out the patient's goals. What are the patient's plans upon discharge from therapy? What does he or she want to be able to do upon discharge from therapy that he or she cannot do at its initiation?

Objective

1. Measure *everything;* avoid estimates and/or terms like "appears" or "functional." All items should be qualified initially in order to show progress when re-evaluated later.

2. Show deficits that require a therapist's skilled care versus that of an aide or a family member. For example, show how your instruction is necessary, evaluate the speed of transfers and the movement of each body part during transfers as well as the assistance needed. Only a PT or OT can work on deviations; an aide can work on mere distance and assistance.

3. Be sure to put a baseline measurement of an activity or deficit in your note if you plan a goal or a treatment that includes that activity.

4. Show significant functional deficits and how objective measurements relate to them.

5. Be careful in reporting mental status. If you are in doubt of a patient's mental status, don't guess, and don't emphasize the negative. A patient may be a little confused but may be able to follow commands well and gain much benefit from therapy. Avoid terms like "confused." If a patient is disoriented as to the date but is oriented to person, place, and task, be specific in what you state. Emphasize the patient's ability to participate in therapy.

6. Use ordinal or ratio scales (e.g., 0–10 or 0–5) to describe objective test results. It is easy for a person reading your notes to understand that 3/5 strength is deficient; "fair" strength does not imply the same level of deficiency unless you are trained. Include copies of rating scales used and/or definitions of terminology particular to your department. Appendix E includes articles with objective rating scales.

7. Don't forget to take vital signs. Gait or transfer training for the sake of endurance is not reimbursable because an aide can ambulate a patient who needs only standby assistance but needs to increase ambulation distance. However, if the heart rate, blood pressure, and/or respiratory rate increases abnormally during ambulation, a therapist's level of skill is needed to further train the patient in ambulation.

8. Re-evaluate and remeasure on a regular basis. It is easier to reset goals and assess the effectiveness of treatment if consistent objective data are available on a regular basis.

Assessment

1. Use specific time estimates for achieving your goals. If goals are not met within an estimated time, explain why, and reset your goals.

2. Explain why a patient's progress may be slower than the usual progress made by patients with the same diagnosis.

3. Goals should
   a. Focus on *the patient* and what he or she will be able to do.
   b. State *the specific behavior* the patient will exhibit.
   c. State any *special conditions* or *equipment* needed or used: assistive devices, types of wraps, prosthetics, orthotics, w/c, and so forth.
   d. Be *measurable* and *include time frames* in which they will be achieved.

4. Explain how deficits (such as strength) relate to function.
5. A clear, concise problem list quickly defines for the reader problems described in more detail in the *O* portion of the note.
6. Be sure to continue to justify treatment as you near the completion of your goals.
7. Point out progress that the patient has made toward the goals as well as further problems needing work.

Planning

1. Include the frequency with which the patient is seen.
2. Be specific enough to describe treatment that requires a therapist versus an aide.
3. Justify the amount of time you spend with the patient by stating the type and amount of treatment the patient receives.

Other

1. Make sure all forms required by the third-party payers are complete and the information required is in the appropriate section and is clear, concise, and easy to find.
2. Attach all notes required by the third-party payers. Keep yourself updated on the frequency of note writing required. Save yourself time by not writing notes any more frequently than they are required; progress is easier to see over a long period of time.
3. For those third-party payers who require preapproval for treatment given, make sure you have preapproval and a preapproval (authorization) number if the organization issues one. Do not exceed the number of preapproved treatment sessions until and unless you obtain preapproval for more treatment.

APPENDIX E

Bibliography

1. Berni, R, Readey, H: PROBLEM-ORIENTED MEDICAL RECORD IMPLEMENTATION: ALLIED HEALTH PEER REVIEW. The CV Mosby Company, St. Louis, MO, 1978.
2. Bernstein, F, et al: "Documentation for Outpatient Physical Therapy." CLINICAL MANAGEMENT. 7(2): 28–30, 1987.
3. Bohannon, RW, Smith, MB: "Interrater Reliability of a Modified Ashworth Scale of Muscle Spasticity." PHYSICAL THERAPY. 67(2): 206–207, 1987.
4. Brunnstrom, S: MOVEMENT THERAPY IN HEMIPLEGIA. Harper and Row, New York, 1970.
5. Daniels, L, Worthingham, C: MUSCLE TESTING TECHNIQUES OF MANUAL EXAMINATION. WB Saunders Co., Philadelphia, 1986.
6. Easton, RE: PROBLEM-ORIENTED MEDICAL RECORD CONCEPTS. Appleton-Century-Crofts, New York, 1974.
7. Feitelberg, SB: THE PROBLEM ORIENTED RECORD SYSTEM IN PHYSICAL THERAPY. University of Vermont, Burlington, VT, 1975.
8. FUNCTIONAL RATING SCALES FOR PHYSICAL THERAPISTS. Documenting Quality Care, Inc., Washington, DC, 1988.
9. Gaidosik, RL, Bohannon, RW: CLINICAL MEASUREMENT OF RANGE OF MOTION. "Review of goniometry emphasizing reliability and validity." PHYSICAL THERAPY. 67(12): 1867–1882, 1987.
10. Griffith, J, Ignatavicius D: THE WRITER'S HANDBOOK: THE COMPLETE GUIDE TO CLINICAL DOCUMENTATION, PROFESSIONAL WRITING AND RESEARCH PAPERS. Resource Applications, Inc., Baltimore, 1986.
11. GUIDE FOR CONDUCT OF THE AFFILIATE MEMBER. American Physical Therapy Association, Alexandria, VA, 1991.
12. GUIDE FOR PROFESSIONAL CONDUCT. American Physical Therapy Association, Alexandria, VA, 1993.
13. GUIDELINES FOR PHYSICAL THERAPY DOCUMENTATION. American Physical Therapy Association, Alexandria, VA, 1993.
14. Gylys, BA, Wedding, ME: MEDICAL TERMINOLOGY: A SYSTEMS APPROACH, 2nd edition. F.A. Davis Company, Philadelphia, 1988.
15. Hill, JR: THE PROBLEM-ORIENTED APPROACH TO PHYSICAL THERAPY CARE. American Physical Therapy Association, Washington, DC, 1977.
16. Hurst, JW, Walker, HK (eds): THE PROBLEM-ORIENTED SYSTEM. Medcom Press, 1972.
17. IEP: INDIVIDUALIZED EDUCATIONAL PROGRAM. WHAT IS IT/HOW DOES IT WORK? Montgomery County Association for Retarded Citizens, Silver Spring, MD, 1978.
18. INSTRUCTIONAL OBJECTIVES. Teaching Improvement Project Systems for Health Care Educators, Center for Learning Resources, College of Allied Health Professions, University of Kentucky, Lexington.
19. Jette, AM (ed): "Functional Assessment of the Elderly." TOPICS IN GERIATRIC REHABILITATION. 1(3): 1986.
20. Jones, P, Oertel, W: "Developing Patient Teaching Objectives and Techniques: A Self-Instructional Program." NURSE EDUCATOR. September-October, 1977, pp. 3–18.
21. Kane RA, Kane RL: ASSESSING THE ELDERLY: A PRACTICAL GUIDE TO MEASUREMENT. DC Heath & Co., Lexington, MA 1981.

22. Keene, JS, Anderson, CA: "Hip Fractures in the Elderly: Discharge Predictions with a Functional Rating Scale." JAMA. 248(5): 564–567, August 6, 1982.

23. Kendall, FP, McCreary ED: MUSCLE TESTING AND FUNCTION. Williams and Wilkins, Baltimore, 1983.

24. Lew, CB: DOCUMENTATION: THE PT'S COURSE ON SUCCESSFUL REIMBURSEMENT. Professional Health Educators, Inc., Bethesda, MD, 1987.

25. Logan, C, Rice, KM: MEDICAL AND SCIENTIFIC ABBREVIATIONS. Lippincott, Philadelphia, 1987.

26. Mahoney, F, Barthel D: "Functional Evaluation: The Barthel index." MD MED J 14:61–65, 1965.

27. Melzach R: "The McGill Pain Questionnaire: Major Properties & Scoring Methods." PAIN. 1: 177–299, 1975.

28. Nelson, AJ: "Functional Ambulation Profile." PHYSICAL THERAPY. 54(10): 1059–1065, 1974.

29. NIA Conference on Assessment. JOURNAL OF AMERICAN GERIATRICS SOC. [reprint] 31:11 & 12, 1983.

30. Payton, OD, Ozer, MN, Nelson, C: PATIENT PARTICIPATION IN PROGRAM PLANNING. F.A. Davis Company, Philadelphia, 1989.

31. Rothstein, J (ed): MEASUREMENT IN PHYSICAL THERAPY. Churchill Livingston, Inc., New York, 1985.

32. Rothstein, JM, Roy, SH, Wolf, SL: THE REHABILITATION SPECIALIST'S HANDBOOK. F.A. Davis Company, Philadelphia, 1991.

33. Simonton, TE: "HCFA's New Medicare Claims Review Criteria Starts November 11." PROGRESS REPORT. American Physical Therapy Association, 17:10, November 1988.

34. STANDARDS OF PRACTICE FOR PHYSICAL THERAPY. American Physical Therapy Association, Alexandria, VA, 1992.

35. Stewart, DL, Abeln, SH: DOCUMENTING FUNCTIONAL OUTCOMES IN PHYSICAL THERAPY. The CV Mosby Company, St. Louis, MO, 1993.

36. Wakefield, JS, Yarnall, SR (eds): IMPLEMENTING THE PROBLEM-ORIENTED MEDICAL RECORD. MCSA, Seattle, WA, 1976.

37. Walter, JB, Pardee, GP, Molbo, DM (eds): DYNAMICS OF PROBLEM-ORIENTED APPROACHES: PATIENT CARE AND DOCUMENTATION. J.B. Lippincott Company, Philadelphia, 1976.

38. Weed, LL: MEDICAL RECORDS, MEDICAL EDUCATION, AND PATIENT CARE. Year Book Medical Publishers, Inc., Chicago, 1971.

39. Weed, LL: "Medical Records, Patient Care and Medical Education." IRISH JOURNAL OF MEDICAL SCIENCE. 6:271–282, 1964.

40. Weed, LL: "What Physicians Worry About: How to Organize Care of Multiple Problem Patients." MODERN HOSPITAL. 110:90–94, 1968.

41. Wolf, S: CLINICAL DECISION MAKING IN PHYSICAL THERAPY. F.A. Davis Company, Philadelphia, 1985.

Using Flow Sheets

The following is an example of a patient case written in three different manners. The first set of notes is written using the traditional SOAP note format. The second set of notes uses the traditional SOAP note format but records some information on a flow sheet. The third set of notes is written on a note form which is a flow sheet. The note form follows the SOAP note format but is used for certain patients with limited problems. It shows the patient's progress in a simple but straightforward manner. Each note format has its advantages and disadvantages. The following three formats are included here for comparative purposes.

Format 1

04-20-95; status as of 1100: INITIAL ASSESSMENT

Dx: Osteoarthritis ® knee; ® total knee replacement 04-19-95.

S: <u>C/o</u>: Pain ® knee of intensity of 8 (0 = no pain, 10 = worst possible pain). <u>Prior level of function</u>: Indep amb c̄ straight cane at home and in public on all surfaces including stairs. Denies previous use of walker or crutches. <u>Home set-up</u>: Lives alone in a house c̄ 4 steps s̄ handrail at entrance. Floor surfaces are carpeting & linoleum s̄ throw rugs. Owns a straight cane only. <u>Pt. goals</u>: To return home indep c̄ a walker upon D/C.

O: <u>Transfers</u>: Sit ↔ stand & supine ↔ sit c̄ min +1 assist. Mat ↔ chair c̄ mod +1 assist. On/off toilet not tested on this date 2° low Pt. endurance. <u>Gait</u>: In // bars 50% PWB ® LE for ~20 ft. x 2 c̄ min +1 assist. Amb on stairs not feasible on this date. <u>Balance</u>: Good in sitting, standing & amb c̄ walker. <u>Endurance</u>: Fair+/Good− on this date. <u>UEs & Ⓛ LE</u>: WNL strength & AROM. ® <u>LE</u>: At least F strength at hip & ankle c̄ WNL AROM; not assessed further at hip & ankle 2° pain; T strength ® quadriceps & hamstrings. AAROM ® knee: prone 20–45°, supine 20–45°, sitting 25–50°. <u>Mental status</u>: Oriented x 3. Follows commands well.

A: <u>Problem List</u>:

1. Dependent transfers
2. Dependent amb
3. ↓ strength ® LE
4. ↓ AROM ® LE
5. ↓ endurance

<u>Long Term Goals</u>:

1. Indep transfers supine ↔ sit, sit ↔ stand, mat ↔ chair, & on/off toilet within 1 wk.

2. Indep walker amb ~100 ft. x 2 on level surfaces & on 4 steps s̄ handrail 50% PWB Ⓡ LE within 1 wk.
3. Indep in home exercise program within 1 wk.
4. AROM Ⓡ knee to 10–90° within 1 wk. to allow Pt. indep ADL & amb.
5. Ⓡ LE strength at least F to allow for indep transfer within 1 wk.

Short Term Goals: All to be achieved in 4 days
1. All transfers c̄ min +1 assist.
2. Walker amb 50 ft. x 2 on level surfaces.
3. Home exercise program c̄ verbal cues only.
4. AROM Ⓡ knee to 20–60°.

Imp: Rehab. potential good. Should be able to achieve Pt.'s goals. Pt. will need stair walker to amb steps at home.
P: BID in dept: Transfer training, gait training progressing to a walker. AAROM & AROM exercises Ⓡ LE, Pt. will be instructed in home exercise program, CPM at B/S, electrical stimulator Ⓡ quadriceps to tolerance.

04-24-95; status as of 1030:
S: C/o: Rates knee pain intensity as 6.
O: Transfers: On/off toilet c̄ mod +1 assist. Mat ↔ chair & supine → sit c̄ min +1 assist. Sit → supine & sit → stand c̄ standby +1 assist. Stand → sit indep. Gait: c̄ stair walker 50% PWB Ⓡ LE ~50 ft. x 2 c̄ standby +1 assist. Balance good c̄ walker, standing or amb. Ⓡ KNEE AROM: Prone 20–60°, supine 20–58°, sitting 23–63°. Home exercise program: Requires verbal cues to perform correctly.
A: All achieved except toilet transfers. Will work toward Long Term Goals until D/C.
P: Cont. c̄ Rx as outlined in note of 04-20-95.

04-27-95; status as of 1400: DISCHARGE SUMMARY
S: C/o: Rates knee pain intensity as 3. Pt. goals: States feels she has achieved her goals.
O: Transfers: Indep sit ↔ stand, supine ↔ sit, chair ↔ mat, & on/off toilet. Amb: Indep c̄ stair walker 50% PWB Ⓡ LE for 120 ft. x 2 & on 4 steps c̄ stair walker. Ⓡ knee AROM: Prone 10–87°, supine 10–87°, sitting 10–90°. Strength Ⓡ LE: F hamstrings and quadriceps & G hip flexors & extensors & in ankle musculature.
A: Long Term Goals: All achieved.
P: D/C PT 2° to D/C of Pt. from Hospital XYZ to home; pt. was indep in home program & given written copy (attached). Seen by PT for 15 Rx sessions.

Format 2

04-20-95; status as of 1100: INITIAL ASSESSMENT
Dx: Osteoarthritis Ⓡ knee; Ⓡ total knee replacement 04-19-95.
S: C/o: Pain Ⓡ knee of intensity of 8 (0 = no pain, 10 = worst possible pain). Prior level of function: Indep amb c̄ straight cane at home and in public on all surfaces including stairs. Denies previous use of walker or crutches. Home set-up: Lives alone in a house c̄ 4 steps s̄ handrail at entrance. Floor surfaces are carpeting & linoleum s̄ throw rugs. Owns a straight cane only. Pt. goals: To return home indep c̄ a walker upon D/C.
O: Transfers: Sit ↔ stand & supine ↔ sit c̄ min +1 assist. Mat ↔ chair c̄ mod +1 assist. On/off toilet not tested on this date 2° low Pt. endurance. Gait: In // bars 50% PWB Ⓡ LE for ~20 ft. x 2 c̄ min +1 assist. Amb on stairs not feasible on this date. Balance: Good in sitting, standing & amb c̄ walker. Endurance: Fair+/good− on this date. UEs & Ⓛ LE: WNL strength & AROM. Ⓡ LE: At least F strength at hip & ankle c̄ WNL AROM; not assessed further at hip & ankle 2° pain; T strength Ⓡ quadriceps & hamstrings. AAROM Ⓡ knee: See attached flow sheet. Mental status: Oriented x 3. Follows commands well.

A: <u>Problem List:</u>
1. Dependent transfers
2. Dependent amb
3. ↓ strength ® LE
4. ↓ AROM ® LE
5. ↓ endurance

<u>Long Term Goals:</u>
1. Indep transfers supine ↔ sit, sit ↔ stand, mat ↔ chair, & on/off toilet within 1 wk.
2. Indep walker amb ~100 ft. x 2 on level surfaces & on 4 steps s̄ handrail 50% PWB ® LE within 2 wks.
3. Indep in home exercise program within 1 wk.
4. AROM ® knee to 10–90° within 1 wk. to allow Pt. indep ADL & amb.
5. ® LE strength at least F to allow for indep transfer within 1 wk.

<u>Short Term Goals:</u> All to be achieved in 4 days
1. All transfers c̄ min +1 assist.
2. Walker amb 50 ft. x 2 on level surfaces.
3. Home exercise program c̄ verbal cues only.
4. AROM ® knee to 20–60°.

<u>Imp:</u> Rehab. potential good. Should be able to achieve Pt.'s goals. Pt. will need stair walker to amb steps at home.

P: BID in dept: Transfer training, gait training progressing to a walker. AAROM & AROM exercises ® LE, Pt. will be instructed in home exercise program, CPM at B/S, electrical stimulator ® quadriceps to tolerance.

04-24-95; status as of 1030:
S: <u>C/o:</u> Rates knee pain intensity as 6.
O: <u>Transfers:</u> On/off toilet c̄ mod +1 assist. Mat ↔ chair & supine → sit c̄ min +1 assist. Sit → supine & sit → stand c̄ standby +1 assist. Stand → sit indep. <u>Gait:</u> c̄ stair walker 50% PWB ® LE ~50 ft. x 2 c̄ standby +1 assist. Balance good c̄ walker, standing or amb. ® <u>KNEE AROM:</u> See attached flow sheet. <u>Home exercise program:</u> Requires verbal cues to perform correctly.
A: All achieved except toilet transfers. Will work toward Long Term Goals until D/C.
P: Cont. c̄ Rx as outlined in note of 04-20-95.

04-27-95; status as of 1400: DISCHARGE SUMMARY
S: <u>C/o:</u> Rates knee pain intensity as 3. <u>Pt. goals:</u> States feels she has achieved her goals.
O: <u>Transfers:</u> Indep sit ↔ stand, supine ↔ sit, chair ↔ mat, & on/off toilet. <u>Amb:</u> Indep c̄ stair walker 50% PWB ® LE for 120 ft. x 2 & on 4 steps c̄ stair walker. ® <u>knee AROM:</u> See attached flow sheet. <u>Strength ® LE:</u> F hamstrings and quadriceps & G hip flexors & extensors & in ankle musculature.
A: <u>Long Term Goals:</u> All achieved.
P: D/C PT 2° to D/C of Pt. from Hospital XYZ to home; Pt. was indep in home program & given written copy (attached). Seen by PT for 15 Rx sessions.

KNEE ROM FLOW SHEET			
	Date: 04-20-95 **Time:** 1100 PT: _____ PROM/AAROM/AROM	**Date:** 04-24-95 **Time:** 1030 PT: _____ PROM/AAROM/AROM	**Date:** 04-27-95 **Time:** 1400 PT: _____ PROM/AAROM/AROM
Knee Flexion			
Prone	45°	60°	87°
Supine	45°	58°	87°
Sitting	50°	63°	90°
Knee Extension			
Prone	−20°	−20°	−10°
Supine	−20°	−20°	−10°
Sitting	−25°	−23°	−10°

Format 3

Name: _____

Pt. #: _____ Room: _____

Dr.: _____ Age: _____

Therapist: _____

Physical Therapy
Progressive Gait Report
Initial Evaluation

| **Dx:** Osteoarthritis Ⓡ knee: Ⓡ THR 04-19-95 | **Date:** 04-20-95 **Time:** 1100 |

SUBJECTIVE: C/o: Pain Ⓡ knee intensity of 8 (0 = no pain, 10 = worst possible pain). <u>Prior level of function:</u> Indep amb c̄ straight cane at home & in public on all surfaces including stairs. Denies previous use of walker or crutches. <u>Home set-up:</u> Lives alone in a house c̄ 4 steps s̄ handrail at entrance. Floor surfaces are carpeting & linoleum s̄ throw rugs. Owns a straight cane only. <u>Pt. goals:</u> To return home indep c̄ a walker upon D/C.

	OBJECTIVE:				
T				**Device:** // bars	
R	Sit → stand	Min + 1		**Wt. bearing:** 10% PWB Ⓡ LE	
A	Stand → sit	Min + 1		**Distance:** ~20 ft. x 2	
N	Supine → sit	Min + 1	**G**	**Assistance:** Min + 1	
S	Sit → supine	Min + 1	**A**	**Deviations:** None noted	
F	Bed/mat → chair	Mod + 1	**I**	**Stairs/1-step:** Not tested	
E	Chair → bed/mat	Mod + 1	**T**	**Balance** **Sit:** Good	
R	On toilet/commode	Not tested		**Stand:** Good in // bars	
S	Off toilet/commode	Not tested		**Walk:** Good in // bars	
				Endurance: Fair +/good−	

EXTREMITIES: UEs & Ⓛ LE: WNL strength & AROM. Ⓡ LE: At least F strength at hip & ankle c̄ WNL AROM; not assessed further at hip & ankle 2° pain; T strength Ⓡ quadriceps & hamstrings. <u>AAROM Ⓡ KNEE:</u> Prone 20–45°, supine 20–45°, sitting 25–50°.

MENTAL STATUS: Oriented x 3. Follows commands well.

ASSESSMENT: **PROBLEM LIST:**	(1) Dependent transfers, (2) dependent amb, (3) ↓ strength Ⓡ LE, (4) ↓ AROM Ⓡ LE, (5) ↓ endurance
P.T. IMP:	Rehab. potential good. Should be able to achieve Pt.'s goals. Pt. will need stair walker to amb steps at home.
LONG TERM GOALS:	Within 1 wk: (1) Indep transfers supine ↔ sit, sit ↔ stand, mat ↔ chair, & on/off toilet. (2) Indep walker amb ~100 ft. x 2 on level surfaces & on 4 steps s̄ handrail 50% PWB Ⓡ LE. (3) Indep in home exercise program. (4) AROM Ⓡ knee to 10–90° to allow Pt. indep ADL & amb. (5) Strength at least F Ⓡ LE to allow for indep transfers.
SHORT TERM GOALS:	Within 4 days: (1) All transfers c̄ min +1 assist. (2) Walker amb 50 ft. x 2 on level surfaces. (3) Home exercise program c̄ verbal cues only. (4) AROM Ⓡ knee to 20–60°.

PLAN: BID in dept: Transfer training, gait training progressing to a walker, AAROM AROM exercises Ⓡ LE, Pt. will be instructed in home program, CPM at B/S, electrical stimulator Ⓡ quadriceps to tolerance.

Name: _____

Pt. #: _____ Room _____

Dr: _____ Age _____

Diagnosis: _____

Physical Therapy
Progressive Gait Report
Interim Updates/Discharge Summary

		Date: 04-24-95 Time: 1030 PT:	Date: 04-27-95 Time: 1400 PT:
S:		Rates knee pain intensity as 6.	Rates knee pain intensity as 3.
O:			
T	Sit → stand	Standby + 1	Indep
R	Stand → sit	Indep	Indep
A	Supine → sit	Min + 1	Indep
N	Sit → supine	Standby + 1	Indep
S	Bed/mat → chair	Min + 1	Indep
F	Chair → bed/mat	Min + 1	Indep
E	On toilet/commode	Mod + 1	Indep
R	Off toilet/commode	Mod +1	Indep
S			
	Device	Stair walker	Stair walker
G	**Wt. bearing**	50% PWB ⓇLE	50% PWB ⓇLE
A	**Distance**	~50 ft. x 2	~100 ft. x 2
I	**Assistance**	Standby + 1	Indep
T	**Deviations**	None noted	None noted
	Stairs/1-step	Not yet tested	Indep
	Balance Sit	Good	Good
	Stand	Good	Good
	Walk	Good	Good
	Endurance	Good −	Good
	Extremities	AAROM Ⓡ knee: Prone 20–60° Supine 20–58° Sitting 23–63°	AAROM Ⓡ knee: Prone: 10–87° Supine 10–87° Sitting 10–90°; strength F in Ⓡ quads & hamstrings & G hip flexors and extensors & in ankle musculature
	Mental status	Unchanged from 04-20-95	Unchanged from 04-20-95
A	**Long term goals**	Not yet achieved; cont. as set on 04-20-95	Achieved
	Short term goals	All achieved except toilet transfers; will work toward long term goals	Achieved
P		Cont. c̄ Rx as outlined in note of 04-20-95	D/C p̄ 15 Rx 2° D/C of Pt. from Hospital XYZ to home; Pt. indep in home program & given written copy (attached)